Thom Garfat
Editor

A Child and Youth Care Approach to Working with Families

A Child and Youth Care Approach to Working with Families has been co-published simultaneously as *Child & Youth Services*, Volume 25, Numbers 1/2 2003.

Pre-publication
REVIEWS,
COMMENTARIES,
EVALUATIONS . . .

"From ethics to data, from activities to support groups, from frontline to being in family homes–IT'S ALL HERE. Child and youth care practitioners, students, and anyone remotely interested in moving beyond just being child-centered to genuinely believing that family must be involved will benefit from reading this book. The benefit comes not only from the importance of the material presented, but from the feeling that the authors have truly been there."

Karl W. Gompf, BSc, MA
Consultant in Child & Youth Care
Red River College
Winnipeg, Manitoba, Canada

More pre-publication
REVIEWS, COMMENTARIES, EVALUATIONS . . .

"IMPORTANT. . . . AN ESSENTIAL REFERENCE for any college or university program committed to professional education and training in this field. There is much to commend in this book, with contributions from professionals working directly with children and young people as well as from others engaged in the education and training of child and youth care workers. It will be of interest to anyone working in the field who wishes to explore new ways of engaging family members as active partners in the care of troubled or troublesome children and young people."

Leon C. Fulcher, PhD, MSW
Professor and Assistant Dean
College of Family Sciences
Zayed University
Abu Dhabi–United Arab Emirates

The Haworth Press, Inc.

A Child and Youth Care
Approach to Working
with Families

A Child and Youth Care Approach to Working with Families has been co-published simultaneously as *Child & Youth Services*, Volume 25, Numbers 1/2 2003.

The *Child & Youth Services*™ Monographic "Separates"

Below is a list of "separates," which in serials librarianship means a special issue simultaneously published as a special journal issue or double-issue *and* as a "separate" hardbound monograph. (This is a format which we also call a "DocuSerial.")

"Separates" are published because specialized libraries or professionals may wish to purchase a specific thematic issue by itself in a format which can be separately cataloged and shelved, as opposed to purchasing the journal on an on-going basis. Faculty members may also more easily consider a "separate" for classroom adoption.

"Separates" are carefully classified separately with the major book jobbers so that the journal tie-in can be noted on new book order slips to avoid duplicate purchasing.

You may wish to visit Haworth's website at . . .

http://www.HaworthPress.com

. . . to search our online catalog for complete tables of contents of these separates and related publications.

You may also call 1-800-HAWORTH (outside US/Canada: 607-722-5857), or Fax 1-800-895-0582 (outside US/Canada: 607-771-0012), or e-mail at:

docdelivery@haworthpress.com

A Child and Youth Care Approach to Working with Families, Thom Garfat, PhD (Vol. 25, No. 1/2, 2003). *"From ethics to data, from activities to support groups, from frontline to being in family homes–it's all here." (Karl W. Gompf, BSc, MA, Consultant in Child and Youth Care, Red River College, Winnipeg, Manitoba, Canada)*

Pain, Normality, and the Struggle for Congruence: Reinterpreting Residental Care for Children and Youth, James P. Anglin (Vol. 24, No. 1/2, 2002). *"Residential care practitioners, planners, and researchers will find much of value in this richly detailed monograph. Dr. Anglin's work adds considerably to our understanding of the residential care milieu as a crucible for change, as well as a scaffolding of support that transects community, child, and family." (James Whitaker, PhD, Professor of Social Work, The University of Washington, Seattle)*

Residential Child Care Staff Selection: Choose with Care, Meredith Kiraly (Vol. 23, No. 1/2, 2001). *"Meredith Kiraly is to be congratulated. . . . A lucid, readable book that presents the fruits of international experience and research relevant to the assessment and selection of child care workers, and which does so in a way that leads to practical strategies for achieving improvements in this important field. This book should be read by anyone responsible for selection into child care roles." (Clive Fletcher, PhD, FBPsS, Emeritus Professor of Occupational Psychology, Goldsmiths' College, University of London; Managing Director, Personnel Assessment Limited)*

Innovative Approaches in Working with Children and Youth: New Lessons from the Kibbutz, edited by Yuval Dror (Vol. 22, No. 1/2, 2001). *"Excellent. . . . Offers rich descriptions of Israel's varied and sustained efforts to use the educational and social life of the kibbutz to supply emotional and intellectual support for youngsters with a variety of special needs. An excellent supplement to any education course that explores approaches to serving disadvantaged children at risk of failing both academically and in terms of becoming contributing members of society." (Steve Jacobson, PhD, Professor, Department of Educational Leadership and Policy, University of Buffalo, New York)*

Working with Children on the Streets of Brazil: Politics and Practice, Walter de Oliveira, PhD (Vol. 21, No. 1/2, 2000). Working with Children on the Streets of Brazil *is both a scholarly work on the phenomenon of homeless children and a rousing call to action that will remind you of the reasons you chose to work in social services.*

Intergenerational Programs: Understanding What We Have Created, Valerie S. Kuehne, PhD (Vol. 20, No. 1/2, 1999).

Caring on the Streets: A Study of Detached Youthworkers, Jacquelyn Kay Thompson (Vol. 19, No. 2, 1999).

Boarding Schools at the Crossroads of Change: The Influence of Residential Education Institutions on National and Societal Development, Yitzhak Kashti (Vol. 19, No. 1, 1998). *"This book* is an essential, applicable historical reference for those interested in positively molding the social future of the world's troubled youth." *(Juvenile and Family Court Journal)*

The Occupational Experience of Residential Child and Youth Care Workers: Caring and Its Discontents, edited by Mordecai Arieli, PhD (Vol. 18, No. 2, 1997). *"Introduces the social reality of residential child and youth care as viewed by care workers, examining the problem of tension between workers and residents and how workers cope with stress." (Book News, Inc.)*

The Anthropology of Child and Youth Care Work, edited by Rivka A. Eisikovits, PhD (Vol. 18, No. 1, 1996). *"A fascinating combination of rich ethnographies from the occupational field of residential child and youth care and the challenging social paradigm of cultural perspective." (Mordecai Arieli, PhD, Senior Teacher, Educational Policy and Organization Department, Tel-Aviv University, Israel)*

Travels in the Trench Between Child Welfare Theory and Practice: A Case Study of Failed Promises and Prospects for Renewal, George Thomas, PhD, MSW (Vol. 17, No. 1/2, 1994). *"Thomas musters enough research and common sense to blow any proponent out of the water. . . . Here is a person of real integrity, speaking the sort of truth that makes self-serving administrators and governments quail." (Australian New Zealand Journal of Family Therapy)*

Negotiating Positive Identity in a Group Care Community: Reclaiming Uprooted Youth, Zvi Levy (Vol. 16, No. 2, 1993). *"This book will interest theoreticians, practitioners, and policymakers in child and youth care, teachers, and rehabilitation counselors. Recommended for academic and health science center library collections." (Academic Library Book Review)*

Information Systems in Child, Youth, and Family Agencies: Planning, Implementation, and Service Enhancement, edited by Anthony J. Grasso, DSW, and Irwin Epstein, PhD (Vol. 16, No. 1, 1993). *"Valuable to anyone interested in the design and the implementation of a Management Information System (MIS) in a social service agency. . ." (John G. Orme, PhD, Associate Professor, College of Social Work, University of Tennessee)*

Assessing Child Maltreatment Reports: The Problem of False Allegations, edited by Michael Robin, MPH, ACSW (Vol. 15, No. 2, 1991). *"A thoughtful contribution to the public debate about how to fix the beleaguered system . . . It should also be required reading in courses in child welfare." (Science Books & Films)*

People Care in Institutions: A Conceptual Schema and Its Application, edited by Yochanan Wozner, DSW (Vol. 14, No. 2, 1990). *"Provides ample information by which the effectiveness of internats and the life of staff and internees can be improved." (Residential Treatment for Children & Youth)*

Being in Child Care: A Journey Into Self, edited by Gerry Fewster, PhD (Vol. 14, No. 2, 1990). *"Evocative and provocative. Reading this absolutely compelling work provides a transformational experience in which one finds oneself alternately joyful, angry, puzzled, illuminated, warmed, chilled." (Karen VanderVen, PhD, Professor, Program in Child Development and Child Care, School of Social Work, University of Pittsburgh)*

Homeless Children: The Watchers and the Waiters, edited by Nancy Boxill, PhD (Vol. 14, No. 1, 1990). *"Fill[s] a gap in the popular and professional literature on homelessness. . . . Policymakers, program developers, and social welfare practitioners will find it particularly useful." (Science Books & Films)*

Perspectives in Professional Child and Youth Care, edited by James P. Anglin, MSW, Carey J. Denholm, PhD, Roy V. Ferguson, PhD, and Alan R. Pence, PhD (Vol. 13, No. 1/2, 1990). *"Reinforced by empirical research and clear conceptual thinking, as well as the recognition of the relevance of personal transformation in understanding quality care." (Virginia Child Protection Newsletter)*

Specialist Foster Family Care: A Normalizing Experience, edited by Burt Galaway, PhD, MS, and Joe Hudson, PhD, MSW (Vol. 12, No. 1/2, 1989). *"A useful and practical book for policymakers and professionals interested in learning about the benefits of treatment foster care." (Ira M. Schwartz, MSW, Professor and Director, Center for the Study of Youth Policy, The University of Michigan School of Social Work)*

Helping the Youthful Offender: Individual and Group Therapies That Work, edited by William B. Lewis, PhD (Vol. 11, No. 2, 1991). *"In a reader-friendly and often humorous style, Lewis explains the multilevel approach that he deems necessary for effective treatment of delinquents within an institutional context." (Criminal Justice Review)*

Family Perspectives in Child and Youth Services, edited by David H. Olson, PhD (Vol. 11, No. 1, 1989). *"An excellent diagnostic tool to use with families and an excellent training tool for our* *family therapy students. . . . It also offers an excellent model for parent training."* (Peter Maynard, PhD, Department of Human Development, University of Rhode Island)

Transitioning Exceptional Children and Youth into the Community: Research and Practice, edited by Ennio Cipani, PhD (Vol. 10, No. 2, 1989). *"Excellent set of chapters. A very fine contribution to the literature. Excellent text."* (T. F. McLaughlin, PhD, Department of Special Education, Gonzaga University)

Assaultive Youth: Responding to Physical Assaultiveness in Residential, Community, and Health Care Settings, edited by Joel Kupfersmid, PhD, and Roberta Monkman, PhD (Vol. 10, No. 1, 1988). *"At last here is a book written by professionals who do direct care with assaultive youth and can give practical advice."* (Vicki L. Agee, PhD, Director of Correctional Services, New Life Youth Services, Lantana, Florida)

Developmental Group Care of Children and Youth: Concepts and Practice, Henry W. Maier, PhD (Vol. 9, No. 2, 1988). *"An excellent guide for those who plan to devote their professional careers to the group care of children and adolescents."* (Journal of Developmental and Behavioral Pediatrics)

The Black Adolescent Parent, edited by Stanley F. Battle, PhD, MPH (Vol. 9, No. 1, 1987). *"A sound and insightful perspective on black adolescent sexuality and parenting."* (Child Welfare)

Qualitative Research and Evaluation in Group Care, edited by Rivka A. Eisikovits, PhD, and Yitzhak Kashti, PhD (Vol. 8, No. 3/4, 1987). *"Well worth reading. . . . should be read by any nurse involved in formally evaluating her care setting."* (Nursing Times)

Helping Delinquents Change: A Treatment Manual of Social Learning Approaches, Jerome S. Stumphauzer, PhD (Vol. 8, No. 1/2, 1986). *"The best I have seen in the juvenile and criminal justice field in the past 46 years. It is pragmatic and creative in its recommended treatment approaches, on target concerning the many aspects of juvenile handling that have failed, and quite honest in assessing and advocating which practices seem to be working reasonably well."* (Corrections Today)

Residential Group Care in Community Context: Insights from the Israeli Experience, edited by Zvi Eisikovits, PhD, and Jerome Beker, EdD (Vol. 7, No. 3/4, 1986). *A variety of highly effective group care settings in Israel are examined, with suggestions for improving care in the United States.*

Adolescents, Literature, and Work with Youth, edited by J. Pamela Weiner, MPH, and Ruth M. Stein, PhD (Vol. 7, No. 1/2, 1985). *"A variety of thought-provoking ways of looking at adolescent literature."* (Harvard Educational Review)

Young Girls: A Portrait of Adolescence Reprint Edition, Gisela Konopka, DSW (Vol. 6, No. 3/4, 1985). *"A sensitive affirmation of today's young women and a clear recognition of the complex adjustments they face in contemporary society."* (School Counselor)

Adolescent Substance Abuse: A Guide to Prevention and Treatment, edited by Richard E. Isralowitz and Mark Singer (Vol. 6, No. 1/2, 1983). *"A valuable tool for those working with adolescent substance misusers."* (Journal of Studies on Alcohol)

Social Skills Training for Children and Youth, edited by Craig LeCroy, MSW (Vol. 5, No. 3/4, 1983). *"Easy to read and pertinent to occupational therapists."* (New Zealand Journal of Occupational Therapy)

Legal Reforms Affecting Child and Youth Services, edited by Gary B. Melton, PhD (Vol. 5, No. 1/2, 1983). *"A consistently impressive book. The authors bring a wealth of empirical data and creative legal analyses to bear on one of the most important topics in psychology and law."* (John Monahan, School of Law, University of Virginia)

Youth Participation and Experiential Education, edited by Daniel Conrad and Diane Hedin (Vol. 4, No. 3/4, 1982). *A useful introduction and overview of the current and possible future impact of experiential education on adolescents.*

Institutional Abuse of Children and Youth, edited by Ranae Hanson (Vol. 4, No. 1/2, 1982). *"Well researched . . . should be required reading for every school administrator, school board member, teacher, and parent."* (American Psychological Association Division 37 Newsletter)

A Child and Youth Care Approach to Working with Families

Thom Garfat

A Child and Youth Care Approach to Working with Families has been co-published simultaneously as *Child & Youth Services*, Volume 25, Numbers 1/2 2003.

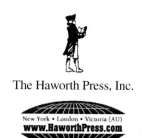

The Haworth Press, Inc.

New York • London • Victoria (AU)
www.HaworthPress.com

A Child and Youth Care Approach to Working with Families has been co-published simultaneously as *Child & Youth Services*™, Volume 25, Numbers 1/2 2003.

The Haworth Press, Inc., 10 Alice Street, Binghamton, NY 13904-1580 USA

Cover design by Marylouise E. Doyle

Library of Congress Cataloging-in-Publication Data

Garfat, Thom.
  A child and youth care approach to working with families / Thom Garfat.
     p. cm.
  "A child and youth care approach to working with families has been co-published simultaneously as Child & Youth Services, Volume 25, Numbers 1/2 2003"–TP Plus.
  Includes bibliographical references and index.
     ISBN 0-7890-2486-1 (hard cover : alk. paper) – ISBN 0-7890-2487-X (soft cover : alk. paper)
  1. Problem children–Institutional care. 2. Problem children–Family relationships. 3. Problem youth–Institutional care. 4. Problem youth–Family relationships. 5. Family social work. 6. Problem families–Services for. I. Child & youth services. Vol. 25, no. 1-2.
  II. Title
  HV713.G375 2004
  362.7–dc22
                                                                          2003027050

Indexing, Abstracting & Website/Internet Coverage

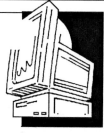

This section provides you with a list of major indexing & abstracting services. That is to say, each service began covering this periodical during the year noted in the right column. Most Websites which are listed below have indicated that they will either post, disseminate, compile, archive, cite or alert their own Website users with research-based content from this work. (This list is as current as the copyright date of this publication.)

(continued)

*Exact start date to come.

(continued)

Special Bibliographic Notes related to special journal issues
(separates) and indexing/abstracting:

- indexing/abstracting services in this list will also cover material in any "separate" that is co-published simultaneously with Haworth's special thematic journal issue or DocuSerial. Indexing/abstracting usually covers material at the article/chapter level.
- monographic co-editions are intended for either non-subscribers or libraries which intend to purchase a second copy for their circulating collections.
- monographic co-editions are reported to all jobbers/wholesalers/approval plans. The source journal is listed as the "series" to assist the prevention of duplicate purchasing in the same manner utilized for books-in-series.
- to facilitate user/access services all indexing/abstracting services are encouraged to utilize the co-indexing entry note indicated at the bottom of the first page of each article/chapter/contribution.
- this is intended to assist a library user of any reference tool (whether print, electronic, online, or CD-ROM) to locate the monographic version if the library has purchased this version but not a subscription to the source journal.
- individual articles/chapters in any Haworth publication are also available through the Haworth Document Delivery Service (HDDS).

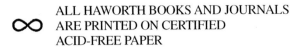

To Henry W. Maier, who has turned so many of us into willing students.

ABOUT THE EDITOR

Thom Garfat, PhD, has been working with troubled young people and their families for over 30 years. He is currently in private practice as a consultant and trainer and has worked with teams, programs, agencies, and governments in Canada, the United States, England, Ireland, Scotland, South Africa, and other countries. Dr. Garfat has developed several residential programs, community-based family intervention programs, family support programs, and numerous other programs for troubled young people and their families. He has worked as a child and youth care worker, a clinical psychologist, and director of a community-based family-intervention program. He also taught child and youth care and family work at the University of Victoria in the School of Child and Youth Care and was Director of treatment for one of Canada's largest group care agencies.

Dr. Garfat is well recognized as a trainer, teacher, consultant, and writer, having published over 100 professional articles on working with youths and families. He is Co-editor of the Canadian journal *Relational Child and Youth Care Practice* and the *International Child Youth Care Network* (CYC-Net)—an Internet-based discussion group and journal. He is a member of a number of child and youth care associations, a member of the Academy of Child and Youth Care Professionals, and is on the board of a number of other journals in the field. His doctoral research at the University of Victoria into the characteristics of helping interventions with troubled youth was awarded the Governor General's Gold Medal. This research has been developed into a training program for child and youth care workers who are engaged with youth and families and has since become a foundation for the field.

A Child and Youth Care Approach to Working with Families

CONTENTS

Foreword

J. K. Rowling's heroes of popular culture, Harry Potter, Hermione Granger and Ron Weasley, provide rich metaphors for contemporary child and youth care practice in the Western world. It is not so much the broomstick games of Quidditch or the images of sorcery that spring to mind so much as the lived experiences of young people leaving childhood and entering adolescence, the transitions from family life to semi-independent living, and the life-space dramas experienced between the worlds of families and the worlds of residential centers. Daily life experiences with these fictional characters have transformed Harry and his friends into household names amongst a whole generation of young people. Few examples can be found in history where young people the world over have waited so eagerly for each new installment or queued in such numbers for each new blockbuster film. Given the opportunity for an early read of chapters that make up this new volume about a child and youth care approach to working with families, it was difficult to avoid making comparisons with challenges illustrated in the fictional world of Harry Potter.

Like Rowling, Garfat and his colleagues have attempted something new, even though it is doubtful whether this volume will sell on a par with Harry Potter. These authors have drawn from direct experiences of working with children, young people, and their families to articulate something that practice wisdom has known for a long time: Families remain important figures in the lives of all children in care. Each of the writers took risks by daring to enter–or even stake claims to–a practice domain carefully guarded by other, more established and reputable professions (if measured by volumes of scholarly prose). Many professions lay claim to the domain of family work, be it family therapy, therapeutic work with families, family casework, or parenting education. However, it is the "magic" that resonates from direct practice experiences with young people and their families that makes this volume special, if only as a beginning attempt to say something about being with and building life-space relationships that continue well after the professional hour, the clini-

[Haworth co-indexing entry note]: "Foreword." Fulcher, Leon. Co-published simultaneously in *Child & Youth Services* (The Haworth Press, Inc.) Vol. 25, No. 1/2, 2003, pp. xix-xxiii; and: *A Child and Youth Care Approach to Working with Families* (ed: Thom Garfat) The Haworth Press, Inc., 2003, pp. xv-xix. Single or multiple copies of this article are available for a fee from The Haworth Document Delivery Service [1-800-HAWORTH, 9:00 a.m. - 5:00 p.m. (EST). E-mail address: docdelivery@haworthpress.com].

cal session, or the therapeutic counselling sessions have finished. The essence of this volume, the magic if you will, is about the practicalities and the importance of forging smart partnerships with mothers, fathers, aunties, uncles, grandparents, foster parents, adopted brothers and sisters, and family members of all shapes and sizes.

Thinking about Harry Potter, it is sometimes surprising to find how many child and youth care workers have never read the books or seen the films! Meanwhile, most of the kids with whom they work can quote whole passages from all five books and identify characters as though they were part of their extended family. In this one might be forgiven for drawing attention to "Muggles" or non-magic folk, like the very family into which Harry Potter was placed as a foster child in kin-group care after the premature death of his parents. That Harry was emotionally and psychologically abused by his Muggle family, indeed even locked in a windowless room under the stairs, might be said to parallel the experiences of many children and young people for whom care and protection services have been established. That Harry learned to express his angry emotions through hurtful wishes may well mirror the thoughts of many a young person, as seen in the example with his nasty cousin at the London reptile centre. And what about the unlikely character of Hagrid, arguably Harry's community "child and youth worker," whose task it was to keep an eye on this unhappy young man until the time came for him to start secondary school at Hogwarts School of Witchcraft and Wizardry? When faced with Hagrid's startling revelations about what made Harry Potter special, Harry's response was not unlike that heard daily by child and youth care workers everywhere: "I'm not a wizard! I'm just Harry!" Or to put it another way, "I'm not special! I'm just . . . (a succession of labels offered by exasperated parents, teachers or professionals)." And with beginning lines just like these, child and youth care workers engage troubled and troublesome kids in their daily living and learning life spaces. That which makes kids special and opens up opportunities for both them and their families is reenacted over and over again with child and youth care workers everywhere. Like magic, the stories continue to unfold.

Those who approach this volume hoping to find new definitions and prescriptions about working with families should look elsewhere. This is not a scholarly tome developed in pursuit of academic citations. This volume is about some of the practicalities of entering into the daily events and patterns of interaction between family members and kids. It is about using daily life events for therapeutic purposes in the life spaces where young people and their families live. It is about the advantages of picking up a dish towel and helping to dry the dishes while interacting with family members about their lived experiences with young people and about the aspirations and dreams that family members hold for their young. It is about rhythms and timing, about connecting with family members and kids in *their* places and times, not just in professional office settings or in a therapeutic group. However, this volume makes no attempt to devalue professional therapeutic activities such as these. Instead, it seeks to complement that which is often missing, in the other 23 hours of each day, or in the other 167 hours of a busy, action-filled week. It is about moving from what Ricks and Bellefeuille called "a knowing" paradigm, driven by expert knowledge, to an ethic of entering into the life-space with the other(s), demonstrating a willingness to walk alongside, or as Shaw and Garfat put it, being where young people and families live their lives. Krueger calls it a way of being in the lived experience with young people and their families, likening the process to modern dance, creating moments of connection, discovery, and empowerment but always wary of the rhythms that connect people so that their interactions have meaning.

Child and youth care workers, like Hagrid–the disgraced wizard and surrogate youth worker at Hogwarts–credibility is earned with young people like Harry Potter and his friends by actually living with them through difficult and scary times. Phelan calls on professional helpers to trust families more and to believe that they know a great deal about what they need or want for their children. All too often, families have been written off as "Muggles" who do not live up to the expectations of those holding "magic wands of authority" or professional expertise. Being with families in their life spaces requires a special kind of magic and what Phelan calls "an observing ego" where one must be continually vigilant about personal boundaries in situations of intimacy. Fewster's primary concern is with the subjective experience of the child or young person, arguing that a child is more than a family member who needs to be acknowledged as a separate and unique being in his or her own right. Charles and Charles caution that there is no one avenue to successful interventions with families.

First interactions do not always go the way one might like. By the time child and youth care workers get involved, many kids and families are jaded by their experiences with helpers, feeling as though the "iron hand of help" may strike again, no matter how desperately they seek an anchor to help them through turbulent times. These practice scholars argue that if change is to occur, it only happens in manageable chunks and through relationships, not interventions. There is no magic wand shop in Diagon Alley where relationships can be exchanged for family-work interventions. And, as VanderVen argues, it is through activities in life spaces that opportunities for new ways of being and interacting are facilitated.

Smith reminds child and youth care readers not to ignore the significant roles played by fathers in the lives of the young people with whom they work. At a time when the dominant discourse challenges patriarchal structures and male dominance in family life, there are institutional forces that exclude fathers and target them as the prevailing source of problems faced by mothers and children. Smith offers a Scottish voice, in this predominantly North American collection, that draws from both direct practice as well as practice research. His conclusions remind the reader that dads are important in their kid's lives. Most men desire to be fathers and to be good fathers as well, often better fathers than they themselves had. Men do not always fulfil as important a role in their children's lives as they would like, and it is easy for professional attitudes and ways of working to label dads as "the problem." Existing services are rarely geared toward supporting dads and may actually discriminate against them. And even though such attitudes may result in practice scholars like Smith being labelled "teachers of the dark arts" at schools like Hogwarts with some, perhaps, arguing that he should be banished to the prisons of Azkaban with other heretics and nonbelievers, it is difficult to dismiss claims that many fathers would welcome support they perceive as credible and non-stigmatising. And, once again, this involves entering into fathers' life spaces and personal rhythms, often using activities to help them learn new ways of being and interacting with their sons and daughters. The reader is left with questions about the meaning of absent dads and what impact absent dads may have on the self-esteem and personal identities of their children.

Both Modlin and McElwee offer practical observations about the processes required to move child and youth care from a history of center-based practice with children and young people removed from their families to working partnerships that give family members a prominent place alongside child and youth care workers in their day-to-day work. Modlin reports on steps taken to involve parents through group home services and, in so doing, to shift the mindsets of child and youth care workers that open new opportunities for all concerned. Writing from an Irish perspective, McElwee traces both historical and policy themes that have prevented families from playing a more active part in social care services in that country. His concerns are about child and youth care workers finding an identity through working with family members in a political environment where other professions seek to draw boundaries around what might be appropriate or about doing the work of others. In the concluding chapter, Hill and Garfat offer valuable insights as a manager and supervisor, arguing that not all child and youth care workers should do work with families, perhaps because they lack maturity and experience. It is especially pleasing to find a supervisor emphasizing the importance of scheduling that supports working with families and reinforcing first priorities about covering the needs of children and young people while making sure to timetable opportunities for family work to happen. It is also fitting that Hill and Garfat remind readers about the economics of child and youth care, pointing to ways in which opportunity cost-benefit arguments might be developed to support child and youth care approaches to working with families.

While there is much to commend in this beginning effort to articulate a child and youth care approach to working with families, it must be said that all the chapters are largely Eurocentric and monocultural in their orientations. It is true that many of the principles identified in this volume might offer insights for child and youth care workers engaging with indigenous families and young people or with children from Hispanic or Afro-Caribbean and Afro-American families. References to culture are few and, where these do appear, they are not developed to any great extent. There is little room for views such as those documented in Rangihau's New Zealand research about child and family welfare services for Maori peoples which found that "at the heart of the matter was a profound misunderstanding or ignorance about the place of a child in Maori society and its relationship with *whanau* (family), *hapu* (sub-tribe), and *iwi* (tribal) structures" (*Puao-te-Ata-tu* [Daybreak] 1986, p. 7). In pursuing family-oriented policies and practices, New Zealand health and welfare workers and teachers–mostly of European ancestry–failed historically to take account of cultural influences that shape the development of indigenous children. Most accept now that, in spite of good intentions, professional efforts with indigenous children in New Zealand as well as in North America and elsewhere have been largely monocultural, where interventions have been informed by ideas imported from elsewhere. Such practices are changing, and some child and youth care workers have gone to great lengths to develop culturally appropriate ways of working with children and families. However, these voices are missing from this volume and will need to be nurtured and supported in future efforts as child and youth care workers continue to articulate more responsive ways of working with indigenous and minority group children and families. Until then, this volume offers an important beginning and is recommended to all concerned with improving child and youth care services, wherever they are.

Leon Fulcher
Zayed University

REFERENCE

Rangihau, J. (1986). Puao-te-Ata-tu (Daybreak): Report of the Ministerial Advisory Committee on a Maori Perspective for the Department of Social Welfare. Wellington: Department of Social Welfare, Government Printing Office, p. 7.

Preface

The head of a federal department quite recently begged a settlement to transform into readable matter a certain mass of material which had been carefully collected into tables and statistics. He hoped to make a connection between the information concerning diet and sanitary conditions, and the tenement house people who sadly needed this information. The head of the bureau said quite simply that he hoped that the settlements could accomplish this, not realizing that to put information into readable form is not nearly enough. It is to confuse a simple statement of knowledge with its application.

Permit me to illustrate from a group of Italian women who bring their underdeveloped children several times a week to Hull House for sanitary treatment, under the direction of a physician. It has been possible to teach some of these women to feed their children oatmeal instead of tea-soaked bread, but it has been done, not by statement at all but by a series of gay little Sunday morning breakfasts given to a group of them in the Hull House nursery. A nutritious diet was then substituted for an inferior one by a social method.

–Jane Addams, 1899
"A Function of the Social Settlements"
[reprinted in Addams, 1992, p. 89]

Jane Addams said that the purpose of the settlement house is to "express the meaning of life in terms of life itself, in forms of activity," and she believed that a settlement works because of reciprocity between its members, even those who are destitute, oppressed, and troublesome.

In 1996, Jerry Beker and I argued that residential care programs in the U.S., based on what we learned about from colleagues in Israel, have few reasons not to practice reciprocity and a social method with youth residents, even difficult youth.

Here, Thom Garfat and his colleagues argue that we have no reason not to practice reciprocity with the parents and families of these same youth. He furthers the work of Addams by illustrating how it is practiced, even with difficult

---

[Haworth co-indexing entry note]: "Preface." Magnuson, Douglas. Co-published simultaneously in *Child & Youth Services* (The Haworth Press, Inc.) Vol. 25, No. 1/2, 2003, pp. xxv-xxvii; and: *A Child and Youth Care Approach to Working with Families* (ed: Thom Garfat) The Haworth Press, Inc., 2003, pp. xxi-xxiii. Single or multiple copies of this article are available for a fee from The Haworth Document Delivery Service [1-800-HAWORTH, 9:00 a.m. - 5:00 p.m. (EST). E-mail address: docdelivery@haworthpress.com].

xxi

parents. And so we have come full circle pedagogically: We cannot practice child and youth care in a way that leaves out the parents nor can we simply blame them for child and youth problems. Reciprocity includes everyone.

Just as Addams challenged preconceptions about immigrants and how persons learn, these authors challenge our preconceptions about parents of difficult children and youth: their capacities, interests, values, and lifestyles. Not only is this a challenge to our own preconceptions about *their* identity. . . . That challenge is also to preconceptions about *our* identity. They challenge us to sustain the primacy of person before behaviors and performance. They challenge us to make ethics a priority over method. They challenge us to practice "care-work" before intervention. They challenge us to place the interpersonal and contextual before the intrapersonal and individual.

Their explication of care-work is timely, because we are nearing the end of a period of naiveté about family work and, it is hoped, the end of a period of dichotomous thinking about families. One choice was to place hope in a range of interventions for families in trouble (e.g., wraparound services, therapy, casework, parent education), but these have not been that successful in either saving money or preventing placement of children outside of the home. Another, earlier choice was to abandon work with the family and to try to save the children. That created new problems between children and families, and it created relationships of hostility and defensiveness between families and care systems.

This dichotomous choice between children and their families was a false, unrealistic choice, and perhaps we may now give it up. Both choices are based on a mistaken hope for the "right" solution and a unitary intervention. Yet the discussions of work with families in these pages makes no false promises of easy success or an easy romanticism about difficult families. What it does promise is a practice of working with families that is consistent with the tradition of child and youth care work, and this book is a good lesson in the pedagogy of that work even for those not interested in family work.

These authors teach us that human development begins with the practices of respect, dignity, and the wholeness of a human life, principles described by Taylor (1989); the child and youth care practice described here begins with this kind of philosophical anthropology of person. There is a basic pedagogical principle here: Like Addams, Garfat argues that parents' dignity is an *a priori* condition and that direct attempts to change them are disrespectful, violates their dignity, and contradicts the inherent, intrinsic organic wholeness of a person's life.

This is not just a principle of family work; it is a guide to all traditional child and youth care work. Development and growth is a mysterious, asynchronous, nonlinear process and dynamic. All child and youth care work aims to further growth and change, yet its pedagogy is not interventionist and direct. Youthwork practice is indirect, cooperative, collaborative, and invitational.

A further characteristic of this paradox is that the reciprocity described in these pages rests on a creative tension between acknowledging the "otherness" of and in clients while nurturing shared experience and common understandings. This is a rich–although demanding–explication of reciprocity and shared experience as alternatives to conformity and similarity, which are the usual standards.

The federal department head, described by Addams, wanted to help and, seeing a linear connection between behavior and problem, asked for a linear intervention. Addams proposed instead a "social method," a nonlinear and moral practice method of respect and dignity.

Here, Garfat and his colleagues have done well in upholding this practice tradition.

Douglas Magnuson

REFERENCES

Addams, J. (1992). *On education.* New Brunswick, NJ: Transaction Publishers.

Beker, J., & Magnuson, D. (1996). *Residential education as an option for at-risk youth.* NY: The Haworth Press, Inc.

Taylor, C. (1989). *Sources of the self: The making of the modern identity.* Cambridge, MA: Harvard.

Introduction

If family ties are to be conserved and family responsibilities insisted upon, systematic attention is needed in dealing with the families of children for whom we are caring. . . . When the child comes into care, the family comes with it. . . .

By such means reconstructive and recreative work with families becomes possible, the child does not stay away from his home any longer than is necessary, and there is ample time for his adjustment and follow-up.

–Carl Carstens, 1927 (quoted in Daniels & Tucker, 1989)

WHAT IS FAMILY?

This collection of papers, from people embedded in the field of child and youth care, is about working with the families of those young people who are sometimes called troubled or troubling. But what is family? This collection does not definitively answer the question. It is, like so many other writings, encompassing of many definitions. It does not, however, avoid the issue.

It would have been nice to start with a clear, singular definition of family, but we find, in our field as in most others, that such a definition is not available. More importantly, a single, common definition would be limiting and restrictive and, quite frankly, it would interfere with effective family work with young people and their families. For young people and families themselves resist any formal definition of what constitutes family, preferring the freedom of a flexible definition.

As you read this collection, you will find, among other, sometimes implied, definitions that family might be:

- The traditional, related group of individuals into which a child is born, which may consist of a few or multiple individuals, close or extended.

All royalties from the sale of this book support *CYC-NET*, an international Website for child and youth care workers [available at www.cyc-net.org].

[Haworth co-indexing entry note]: "Introduction." Garfat, Thom. Co-published simultaneously in *Child & Youth Services* (The Haworth Press, Inc.) Vol. 25, No. 1/2, 2003, pp. 1-6; and: *A Child and Youth Care Approach to Working with Families* (ed: Thom Garfat) The Haworth Press, Inc., 2003, pp. 1-6. Single or multiple copies of this article are available for a fee from The Haworth Document Delivery Service [1-800-HAWORTH, 9:00 a.m. - 5:00 p.m. (EST). E-mail address: docdelivery@haworthpress.com].

- A nonbiologically related group of individuals, living together in a systemically related commitment.
- The individuals to whom the child is attached and who hold a place of primary importance for the young person, but with whom the young person is not living, and with whom the young person may even have limited contact.

We recognize that there are legal, organizational, and functional definitions that have various implications for our work with the young person. But in the end any and all of these definitions seem to be of lesser importance in direct practice with young people and their families. As a field, we appear to have adopted the position that the family is whatever it is as created, determined, and experienced by the young person and the significant others in the young person's life. This "constructed family" is what is most important in our work because it is what is most important to the youth's experiencing.

This is not to suggest disrespect for those other, more formal definitions. Nor does it imply that we ignore, for example, the biological family in favor of the constructed family. Indeed, we often work with a young person and the young person's family to help them have experiences that may change their perception of what constitutes family, thereby modifying perhaps the constructed definition.

I remember a young person who came to stay in a residential center where I was working. On her arrival, we were clearly informed that she "had no family": no parents, no extended relatives, no one. I remember, too, when she left the center. By then she had regular, if infrequent, visits with a distant aunt who had been tracked down and engaged by a persistent staff team. She had regular, more frequent, visits with a man who, while unrelated by blood, had been there at some significant early moments in her development and who was interested in playing some supportive role in her life. She developed close and personal relationships with two other young women, and the three of them decided that they were sisters. In short, when she came, she had no family. When she left, she had some.

Ten years later, as I write this, those connections–that family–still exists. This young person, with the help of a caring staff team, had developed her own family, and her constructed family is as supportive, important, and powerful as any other family might be in the life of a young person. One day I asked her about this constructed family and how she thought of it relative to more traditional families. Her reply was clear enough: "It feels like my family so it is my family."

So in the end, this collection has nothing to offer by way of a clear definition of family. You will find multiple descriptions and definitions. As

Niall McElwee says, "The family today looks very different than it did a couple of decades ago" and, as a result, we need, to quote Grant Charles and Holly Charles, a more "fluid definition of family." Perhaps we would be wisest to align ourselves with Gerry Fewster's interest in the family "as a subjective reality that is constructed collectively and experienced individually" which seems appropriate as child and youth care moves towards a more phenomenological orientation. For when we position ourselves inside the constructed world of the child, we at least position ourselves to attend to the family as experienced by the child and, in the end, maybe that is the only definition that is relevant.

I remember once talking to a young woman about family and what it was for her. She was a young woman who had, like so many of the young people with whom we work, constructed her own family out of the myriad of people who had been a part of her life.

"Family," she said, "is where you belong, isn't it?"

Or the other young person who, when asked, looked at me strangely and replied,"Family is, well, it's the place where your heart feels safe."

In the end, maybe that is a good a definition as any: "Family is the place where you have a sense of belonging and feel safe," for belonging and safety are certainly among the most basic of needs. As the young people implied in the quotes above, family is, more than anything, a feeling, an experience, an experience of self in a particular context. As we explore this territory, as we place ourselves in the position of being with the young person and family, we open the opportunity to know a little more of their experiential world.

YOUTH CARE, YOUTH WORK, CHILD AND YOUTH CARE: WHAT'S IN A NAME?

The reader will also notice that in this collection there is no clear label or name for members of the staff we discuss. In some papers you will find the use of the term Child Care Worker, in others the term Child and Youth Care Worker. At times you will discover the term Youth Worker, and at times, Youth Care Worker, Youth Family Worker, Care Worker or, even, Social Care Worker. Sometimes the label, whatever it is, is capitalized. Sometimes it is not. We have made no attempt here to come to an agreement on one particular term. If the field itself cannot do it, we would be foolish to attempt to do so ourselves (see McElwee & Garfat, 2003). What is important is who we are talking about, not what they are called.

We are talking about those people who work with troubled (well, sometimes not) young people who sometimes live in group care (but not always), and/or are in the care of the system (well, most often anyway). Maybe the easiest thing to say, for the moment, is that we are talking about the direct care, front-line helpers whose positions and work grew out of the influences of the 1950s and 1960s. We see the influences, for example, of Redl and Wineman (1951, 1952), Meyer (1958), Redl (1959), Burmeister (1960), Maier (1957, 1960, 1979), Polsky (1962), Trieshman (see Trieshman, Whittaker, & Brendtro, 1969), Beedell (1970), Beker (1972), and others who work in a variety of environments. For a description of many of those locations of work, the reader is referred to the general literature of the field (e.g., Denholm, Ferguson, & Pence, 1993; McElwee & Garfat, 2003).

Or maybe it is best to say nothing at all because the people for whom this collection was written know exactly who they are. Labeling them with a common definition feels too much like trying to come up with a common definition of the family. The reality is that we who work in this field share much in common and are, ourselves, comfortable with the variety of names, labels, and definitions by which we refer to ourselves. In the end, the variety reflects our collectively constructed and individually experienced identity.

A LITTLE HISTORY BEFORE WE BEGIN

There was a time in our professional history when the family was not seen in a positive light. Indeed, in the early days of our field, family was considered irrelevant (Fewster & Garfat, 1993). Then when it did become relevant, it was negatively so, in that the family was seen as a problem, the enemy, the cause of all this pain and suffering of the child (Garfat & McElwee, 2001). To make this statement is not a criticism of earlier programs or approaches for, indeed, those programs and approaches simply reflected the prevailing attitude of the times (Charles, 2003). We have now, to a great extent, arrived at a place where we see family as a partner, a solution, a way of helping the young person who remains our focus (Garfat & McElwee, 2001). But it is not just the involvement of families that has changed in child and youth care. There have been, as well, dramatic changes in the focus of our work, the role of child and youth care workers and, most important, in the locations in which we work. As you read this collection of writings, you will recognize many of the new roles for child and youth care workers, especially in the community. Child and youth care work has become, finally, a true support to families. In a recent article, Niall McElwee and I summarized the changes over the years in a simple chart, which is offered here as a quick reference (see Table 1). Readers interested in further details could consult the original article.

Suffice to say that in contemporary child and youth care practice, family is the focus (Garfat, 2002). There is an increasing expectation on the part of families, other professionals, and society in general that family will be involved in the care and treatment of young people. For many of us, as Mark Hill says, it is

TABLE 1. Changes in Family Involvement and Work in Child and Youth Care Work

Era Variable	Beginning	Past	Recent/Future
Definition of client and location of problem	child	child/parents	family
Perception of parent and purpose of contact	irrelevant; the enemy; ⎯⎯	parental incompetence; ⎯⎯	person/individual as a part of systems; ⎯⎯
	blaming; information sharing	program input; education; support	collaboration, relationship, intervention into daily life
Role of family members	none, occasional visitor	parenting, contact, input into IIP, recipient of support	client, co-helper, input into daily decision-making
Role of Youth Care Worker	control, protection of child from parents; substitute parents	protection, parent educator, behaviour change, connection	engagement, family interventionist, outreach, facilitation
Location of service	none for parents	in program, community	in home, community and program

Reprinted from Garfat, T. & McElwee, N. (2001). The changing role of family in child and youth care practice. *Journal of Child and Youth Care Work,* 16, 236-248.

difficult now "to imagine how concentrating solely on one family member will lead to lasting change."

Child and youth care in both theory and practice has now placed family as central to effective helping. It is hard to imagine anymore a collection of writing about helping young people that does not include an emphasis on family. It was not that long ago, however, that a collection such as this would have seemed like a radical idea. Now, we hope, it just makes sense.

Thom Garfat

REFERENCES

Beedell, C. (1970). *Residential life with children.* London: Routledge & Kegan Paul.
Beker, J. (1972). *Critical incidents in child care: A case book for child care workers.* New York: Behavioral Publications.
Burmeister, E. (1960). *The professional houseparent.* New York: Columbia University Press.

Charles, G. (in press). Child and youth care in North America: History, issues and changes. In P. Share & N. McElwee (Eds.), *Social care in Ireland*. Dublin: IASCE.

Daniels, J., & Tucker, O. (1989). Transforming the child care institution into a family-oriented system. In *Group care of children: Transitions toward the year 2000*. Washington, DC: Child Welfare League of America.

Denholm, C., Ferguson, R., & Pence, A. (Eds.). (1993). *Professional child and youth care practice*: New York: The Haworth Press, Inc.

Fewster, G., & Garfat, T. (1993). Residential child and youth care. In C. Denholm, R. Ferguson, & A. Pence (Eds.), *Professional child and youth care* (2nd ed., pp. 9-36). Vancouver, BC: University of British Columbia Press.

Garfat, T. (Aug. 2002) *On the development of family work in residential programs*. Available on-line at *www.cyc-net.org*

Garfat, T., & McElwee, N. (2001). The changing role of family in child and youth care practice. *Journal of Child and Youth Care Work, 15-16*, 236-248.

Maier, H. W. (1957). Routines: A pilot study of three selected routines and their impact upon the child in residential treatment. *American Journal of Orthopsychiatry, 27*(3), 701-709.

Maier, H. W. (1960). Essential ingredients for the care and treatment of children in child care institutions. *Proceedings of the third annual conference of the Nebraska conference on child care* (pp. 1-16). Nebraska Psychiatric Institute.

Maier, H. W. (1979). The core of care: Essential ingredients for the development of children at home and away from home. *Child Care Quarterly, 8*(3), 161-173.

McElwee, N., & Garfat, T. (2003). What's in a name?: Exploring title designations. *Irish Journal of Applied Social Science, 4*(1), 5-20.

Meyer, M. (1958). *A guide for child care workers*. New York: Child Welfare League of America.

Polsky, H. (1962). *Cottage six*. Huntington, NY: Krieger Publishing.

Redl, F. (1959). Strategy and technique of the life-space interview. *American Journal of Orthopsychiatry, 29*, 1-18.

Redl, F., & Wineman, D. (1951). *Children who hate: The disorganization and breakdown of behavior controls*. New York: Free Press.

Redl, F., & Wineman, D. (1952). *Controls from within: Techniques for the treatment of the aggressive child*. New York: Free Press.

Trieshman, A. E., Whittaker, J. K., & Brendtro, L. K. (1969). *The other twenty-three hours: Child care work with emotionally disturbed children in a therapeutic milieu*. New York: Aldine de Gruyter.

Working with Families:
Developing a Child
and Youth Care Approach

Thom Garfat

SUMMARY. Recently there has been discussion of a distinctly "youth care approach" to working with families. There are some assumptions of this kind of work, including (a) family life is lived in "daily events," and in those daily life events there are patterns of interacting; (b) child and youth care workers are involved with families as they live their lives; and (c) child and youth care utilizes daily life events for therapeutic purposes, as they occur. Family work interventions are characterized by caring for the family and individual family members, related to the immediate and the overall context, and reflect a way of connecting that fits each family, including their rules, roles, culture, rhythm, timing, and style. *[Article copies available for a fee from The Haworth Document Delivery Service: 1-800-HAWORTH. E-mail address: <docdelivery@haworthpress.com> Website: <http://www.HaworthPress.com> © 2003 by The Haworth Press, Inc. All rights reserved.]*

KEYWORDS. Youthwork with families, youth care work, social work with families, family-centered residential care, child and youth care, family services, family support, parent education, residential care work and families

---

Thom Garfat is affiliated with TransformAction Consulting & Training, Montreal, Quebec, and is Co-editor of *CYC-Net* (www.cyc-net.org) and *Relational Child and Youth Care Practice*.

[Haworth co-indexing entry note]: "Working with Families: Developing a Child and Youth Care Approach." Garfat, Thom. Co-published simultaneously in *Child & Youth Services* (The Haworth Press, Inc.) Vol. 25, No. 1/2, 2003, pp. 7-37; and: *A Child and Youth Care Approach to Working with Families* (ed: Thom Garfat) The Haworth Press, Inc., 2003, pp. 7-37. Single or multiple copies of this article are available for a fee from The Haworth Document Delivery Service [1-800-HAWORTH, 9:00 a.m. - 5:00 p.m. (EST). E-mail address: docdelivery@haworthpress.com].

Digital Object Identifier: 10.1300/J024v25n01_02

It is an early spring weekday evening. John, a youth care worker, is in the family kitchen talking with a father and son about fly-tying. The boy, Bobby, aged 14, is being considered for placement in a residential treatment center. He is under consideration because he keeps getting into fights and thrown out of school. Then the fights carry on at home. After a while he was doing whatever he wanted at home.

A younger brother and sister are in the adjoining living room, bickering while playing a game, their volume gradually rising. Mom is in the bedroom taking a nap. She was napping when the worker arrived. After a few minutes the mom comes screaming out of the bedroom, yelling at the bickering siblings that they should "shut up," her volume overpowering theirs. Mom glances over and notices that the worker is there. She turns back to the other children and continues, without changing volume, intensity, or style.

She yells at them that she has had a tough day and, that if they cared about her, they would be quiet. They stare at her in silence. She then walks into the kitchen, says to her husband, "God, can't you keep them quiet while I am resting?"

Dad retorts: "How was I to know they'd wake you up? They were only playing, you know."

"They were fighting, for God's sake," she responds, and turns to put on the coffee pot.

The worker says, "Evening, Jane," and turns back to the father and son who are both staring at the mom. The father has an angry look on his face. The son looks embarrassed. The worker turns back to the dad and Bobby gets up and goes outside. Mom brings the cups to the table.

We read this scenario and give it meaning. From within our own framework, we critique, judge, and evaluate. We make assumptions. We interpret. We try to make sense out of what we have read. We wonder how the worker is interpreting what is going on and how to respond. In this process some of our assumptions become evident. Our perceptual frame (Bruner, 1990) is partially revealed.

As you read, a number of questions might come to mind:

1. Why are they in the house rather than an office? And why the kitchen?
2. Why are the worker, father, and son talking about flyfishing instead of talking about the youth's difficulties in school or with his parents?
3. What is the meaning of the mother being asleep while the worker, dad, and youth are talking?
4. Why is it that mom's volume, intensity, and style do not change when she sees the worker sitting in the kitchen?
5. Why is the worker not intervening with the siblings?
6. Why did the worker not ask the mother to join them?

7. Does it matter that it is spring?
8. What should the worker do at this point?

The answer to questions like these–and there are many others which might come to mind–depend on a worker's values, beliefs, and orientation toward work with the families of troubled youth. Therefore, before discussing what the worker actually did, I want to look at what it means to work with families from a child and youth care perspective, because such a perspective, indeed a child and youth care approach, is different than other forms of working with families. It is different because it is based on the child and youth care orientation towards change which, in turn, is based on certain assumptions about helping and the helping process. Rather than answer the above questions directly I need to articulate first some of the assumptions that are inherent in a child and youth care approach, identify some of the elements associated with effective interventions, and then identify a process for intervention that is consistent with these.

Throughout this paper, exercises are included which are intended to assist the reader in becoming more familiar with and involved in the principles inherent in this approach.

THREE ASSUMPTIONS OF THE CHILD
AND YOUTH CARE APPROACH

Assumption I:
Family Life Is Lived in "Daily Events,"
and in Those Daily Life Events There Are Patterns of Interacting

Families are an organized manner of living life together. In families we wake, eat, interact, love, raise children, and develop our lives in a myriad of other ways. While it might seem sometimes that the daily events of the families with whom we work are filled with drama, the reality is that, like most of us, the majority of their days are filled with everyday events. Also, like the rest of us, their lives are lived in patterned ways–habitualized ways of interacting with each other and the world in which they live (Minuchin, 1978; Ricks and Garfat, 1989).

So in the opening scenario we see a dramatic interaction. A calm moment erupts in raised voices and stunned responses. Chances are that if there is a consistent pattern here, we would also find it in other areas of this family's life. For if we eliminate the immediate content, what do we see?

Father and son are interacting, albeit with the assistance of a facilitator. Mom is uninvolved at the moment. The two siblings are creating their own distraction. Dad is uninvolved with that. Mom is drawn in by the activity of the two siblings and interprets their activity as a message of not caring about her.

Mom then joins dad and they argue about the two siblings. Simplified, the interpretation is: Mom and dad are uninvolved with each other, and the siblings create a dynamic for them to be involved.

> *Exercise I: Imagine that this is a pattern of daily living or interaction with this family. What are some of the other ways that this pattern might show up in other, less dramatic, places?*

This is one of the things that child and youth care workers do in working with families. They see an interaction and ask if it is typical of this family's way of living life, and then they search for information that might confirm or deny this speculation. In doing this, the child and youth care worker is not looking to make a *diagnosis*. Rather, the worker is seeking to *understand* how the family lives out its life.

In the exercise above, for example, we might speculate that this pattern would show up in a less dramatic way when dad is in the garage working on his hobby, mom is in the kitchen, and one of the siblings falls off his bike and starts to cry. Mom may be drawn from the house, dad drawn from the garage, and they can talk about whether or not the child is hurt. Not dramatic, but the same pattern appears to be there. A child draws the couple together.

This is not to suggest that in any given family there is only one pattern, for in all families there are many. In this family, for example, there may be patterns relating to how mom gets dad involved in caring about her interests or in how the son, Bobby, gets his dad's attention or in how the dad and the other siblings arrange to not be involved with each other.

There are numerous patterned ways of interacting in every family. The task for the helper is to discover and help to change a pattern which might impact on how the family maintains the role of the troubled child, the identified patient, their own troubles, or even how much pain and confusion they have in their lives.

Assumption II:
Child and Youth Care Workers Are Involved with Families as They Live Their Lives

Child and youth care is about intervening within the ordinary way of living of families. It is based on the belief that if people change how they live and interact together–how they are together–they can and will live lives of less pain and greater satisfaction. In order to work this way, child and youth care has chosen to be with families in the environment where they live their lives. This may involve being with families in their home, in the community as they deal with external systems like the schools, in the garden as they do spring planting, in the park while they are out together for pleasure, or any other place where their life is lived. In this statement, as in the previous assumption, we see the connection between a child and youth care approach to working with youth and a child and youth care approach to working with families.

Given that families live their lives in patterns, it is important that the child and youth care worker who wants to help a family modify how they live together will want to be with the family in those times and places where their life is lived–where those patterns show themselves. While people still live out their patterns and dynamics in any environment in which they find themselves (Garfat, 1998; Minuchen, 1978), they normally live their lives in their world, not the world of an office or a counseling room. I know that some people make an argument that when you meet with families in an office, you are meeting in "neutral territory" where the normal clues and triggers associated with their actions are not present. By meeting in "neutral territory," so the argument goes, the helper and family are more free to explore new ways of being, unencumbered by the influences of daily living. There are, however, some specific advantages to being with people where they live their lives. Some of these include:

1. You are able to make direct observations about what is happening rather than having to rely on reported interpretations about what did happen. You experience their life rather than just hear about it.
2. You are able to enter into their life and rhythms.
3. You have multiple opportunities for developing connectedness and relationship.
4. You are helping them experience new interactions in the environment within which those interactions occur. The cues that become associated with the new way of interacting are the cues of their natural environment and not of a neutral territory.
5. They experience you as coming to help them–as reaching out to them– rather than them having to reach out to you.
6. You are more likely to encounter all the family members when you are in their environment than when you ask them to come to your environment.

   Like all assumptions about models of practice, this one is based on certain values, beliefs, and experiences. Ultimately, of course, one makes choices about what to believe about helping, about how change occurs, and about the role and place of the child and youth care worker. One may have certain values around privacy that would suggest that being involved directly in the daily lives of families is intrusive, and thus one might find this approach distasteful. Or one might hold certain values about security, neutrality, or even helping that would suggest this approach does or does not "fit" for the individual worker.

> *Exercise II: Identify some of the values and beliefs that you hold,*
> *the assumptions underlying these, and how they might affect your*
> *commitment to this child and youth care approach of being with families.*

When we look to our values and beliefs and the assumptions which underlay them, we are exploring the territory of self and self in relationship (Fewster, 1990). It is sometimes useful for us to know where these have come from in our own lives because, in knowing this, we are more able to know how it is that we are having the experience we are having at any given point in time (Garfat, 1992, 1994). One of the characteristics of effective child and youth care is that the worker possesses an "active self-awareness" (Garfat, 1998, Ricks, 1989). Knowing about self is essential to being an actively self-aware helper.

In the previous exercise you may have noticed that you have a value about privacy that is something like "parent issues should be kept separate from the children." In exploring the implications of this you may find that you are concerned that working with families in their home may increase the possibility that the children will become more aware of their parents' issues. You may, if you are with families in their natural environment like the one described in the opening scenario to this chapter, find that you are anxious and nervous that the parents may accidentally blurt out some of their own business. You may find yourself focused more on this anxiety than on the interactions of the family members. Notice how this would affect the quality of your work.

On further exploration you may find that this is connected to your own family of origin and some of your own experience. Notice that this is your own experience and not this family's experience. While you may hold this value, this family may not. In order to work effectively, we need to understand the difference. If you want to work in the natural environment of families, you need to know what you believe because beliefs influence action (Ricks, 1989).

Assumption III:
Child and Youth Care Utilizes Daily Life Events for Therapeutic Purposes, as They Occur

This assumption brings us to the heart of the child and youth care approach to working with troubled families. It is within daily life events, in the small, seemingly unimportant moments, where we find the opportunities to help families live their lives differently (Fox, 1995; Garfat, 1998; Maier, 1987; Redl, 1959). Ultimately, this is the goal of a child and youth care approach to working with families: to help family members live their lives differently. We use these naturally occurring opportunities (Peterson, 1988) to help people learn how to do things differently, how to be together differently, and how to interact in a healthier, less painful manner. Look back to the opening scenario of this chapter. Depending on the lens (Ricks, 1989) through which you create your understanding of how families and individuals change, you will find a myriad of opportunities to intervene. Some of them might include:

1. Asking the father to help the mother as she comes from the bedroom.
2. Processing mom's reaction with her.
3. Making the coffee yourself.
4. Telling a story.
5. Sitting on the porch.
6. Talking to the couple about the tension between them.
7. Reflecting out loud on the mother's interpretation of the sibling's behavior.

> *Exercise III: What are the opportunities for intervention that you see in the scenario as described? What makes that an opportunity for you?*

As I discussed, the focus of our intervention is not just on those dramatic interactions. When we find patterns and we see how they also occur in less dramatic moments, we also find the opportunity for intervention. If you look at the other places in which the same pattern might occur, you will see that these are also opportunities, because the same dynamic is occurring there as in the more dramatic interactions. There are specific reasons why it might be better to intervene in those less dramatic moments.

1. In less dramatic moments, people are less emotional and more able to reflect on–and be "in touch with" their experience of–what is happening and the connections between this moment and others.
2. In calmer moments of interaction people are less likely to feel the need to defend against your observations.
3. In calmer moments the helper might be more focused on the dynamic and less on personal anxiety.

There are other reasons, of course, why an intervention in a less dramatic interaction is sometimes preferable, but the above three are sufficient to make the point. In allowing ourselves to focus on less dramatic moments we increase the range of opportunities available to us to be helpful. The goal of our work is not to be a therapy but to be therapeutic. The child and youth care worker is therapeutic but is not a therapist.

Based on these three assumptions then, the child and youth care worker engages with families. While the foregoing has suggested something about where and why the worker might intervene, it has not addressed the question of the characteristics of those interventions. Recent research (Garfat, 1998) has suggested that it is possible to identify characteristics associated with effective child and youth care interventions. The following section translates those characteristics into the territory of child and youth care work with families.

SOME CHARACTERISTICS OF CHILD AND YOUTH CARE INTERVENTION WITH FAMILIES

As suggested in the foregoing section, the child and youth care intervention can be defined partially by the location of the intervention (i.e., where families live their lives) and in the focus of the intervention (into their patterns of daily living). It would also appear that there are some specific characteristics to those interventions when they are consistent with the child and youth care approach. This section identifies and elaborates on some of those characteristics which are, in the author's experience, related to effective child and youth care work.

Interventions are Characterized by Caring for the Family and Individual Family Members

Child and youth care work is a relationship-based form of helping (Fewster, 1990; Fox, 1995; Garfat, 1998; Krueger, 1998) that is based on a sense of caring for and about others. Within the context of a child and youth care approach, caring is defined in terms of action (Ricks, 1992). Thus, the expression of caring is seen in the actions of the helper in relationship with the family and family members. As Austin and Halpin (1989) pointed out, there are certain conditions under which a caring response is likely to occur and from this it is possible to identify some of the characteristics of a caring intervention (action). According to them a caring intervention is one which:

- values other(s),
- respects the authenticity of other(s),
- reflects a view of other(s) as subject, not object,
- demonstrates a belief that other(s) can be helped,
- is adapted to the needs of others when appropriate, and
- is undertaken as an end to itself.

This list of characteristics, while far from exhaustive, serves to demonstrate the complexity of the caring response in interventions with families, because in all cases there is more than one person to be taken into consideration. It is far simpler, for example, to undertake a caring intervention when one only has to be concerned with the impact of one's actions on the youth, but it becomes much more complex when we must also consider the impact of the intervention or action on the child, siblings, and both parents, with perhaps a grandparent or extended family member added in for extra confusion. In working with families, our "client" is the family, not just the youth and, therefore, our interventions must demonstrate a caring for all.

It is also complicated by our tendency to objectify people because of their actions and how we interpret those actions: He is the aggressor, she is the martyr, he is an inadequate parent, she is a problem, they are a dysfunctional family. When we label people in this manner, we stop relating to them as humans, as real people with real pain and real needs. When we stop relating to them as real people, we cannot manifest caring.

Exercise IV: Identify the characteristics of individuals or families for whom it would be difficult for you to offer a caring response.

Caring is not a strategy or a technique evoked at the appropriate moment in working with families. It is a basic way of being, of operating in the world. It is something that evolves developmentally as we move through life, just as the other aspects of our selves evolve. One cannot go to a short course to learn how to care. However, if one is a caring person and one cares about families and individual family members, one can choose how to express that caring.

What counts as caring for one person may, for another person, not be considered as an expression of caring. Thus in our work with families, we need to learn and to come to understand what counts as caring for each of the individuals in the family. It is only in this way that we can construct interventions that may be experienced as caring by all. The following story demonstrates this idea.

> In the late 1980s, I had the opportunity to run a residential treatment centre for adolescents. Part of my role was to interview families at the point of intake of the youth into the program. Mary and her mother showed up one early morning for a scheduled intake. During our meeting, I asked the mother how she felt about placing Mary in the program. Her response was, "I feel good about it. I was here when I was her age and it really helped me. I hope that it is going to help her the same. I'm doing it because I'm worried about what she's doing and I care about what happens to her."

You can probably predict Mary's response: "If you really cared about me, you would let me go stay with Dad. You're putting me here because you just want to get rid of me."

All actions are interpreted through the perceptual frame of each individual, according to Bruner (1990). We make meaning of things in our own way. What counts as caring for you, the helper, may not count as caring for the family. In general, however, if we structure our interventions according to the characteristics of a caring response, we have a better chance of having our actions experienced as caring.

> *Exercise V: Identify what counts as caring for you. What are the gestures, actions, statements, and style characteristics that you associate with caring? What are some actions others might consider to be caring that would not be interpreted as caring by you?*

For each person these will probably vary, just as they will for each family member. In adapting our presentation and actions to fit the needs of the individual family members, we demonstrate our caring about them.

The Intervention Is Related to the Immediate and Connected to the "Overall"

Child and youth care work is about being with the other in the present moment, living life as it is happening in the current context (Fewster, 1990; Kruger, 1991, 1998), while bearing in mind that what we are experiencing with a family at any given moment probably reflects a patterned way of being. It is not about what happened last week, although sometimes that may appear to be the content of an interaction, but rather about what is happening at this moment as we interact together. Interventions that are effective are related first to the immediate action and connected to the overall goals, not about previous events (Garfat, 1998). There are a number of reasons why this might make sense:

1. Interventions addressed to the immediate are addressed to the person's or family's current experience or experiencing.
2. When we address the immediate, there has not been time to recreate the experience through the distortions of time.
3. When we deal with the immediate, we are able to benefit from direct observations of the interactions. Rather than addressing other's interpretations of those interactions, we make our own. We deal with what people did, rather than with what they said they did.
4. When we deal with the immediate, we are in the present with other as the experience is occurring. The opportunity is there, then, for us to enter into the experience together with the other, what some have called "joint experiencing" (Garfat, 1998; Krueger, 1998; Peterson, 1988).

Dealing with the immediate places a high demand on the child and youth care worker. It requires a high level of cognitive activity while, at the same time, the emotional experience of the worker may also be demanding or distracting. Being in the present does not allow time for reflective consideration from a distance as might be the case when we are dealing with something that happened yesterday or last week. At the same time, for example, that the child and youth care worker is experiencing anxiety about what is going to happen or having to separate self from other, it is also necessary to be connecting the present activity to an overall understanding of the family. This is the key to structuring effective interventions with families from a child and youth care perspective: connecting the immediate interaction to the patterns of living which are the overall focus of the work with this particular family. Let me try to illustrate through a story.

Imagine a family, the Davids, in which the two adults have, for whatever reason, moved out of intimacy over the past number of years. They find that they have little about themselves that they are able to talk about with each other. Like many couples in this situation they have taken to talking, when they do, about other things: the weather, the house, and, especially, the children. Talking about the children is safe territory because it involves talking about the other rather than self.

The worker has observed, through being with the family in their home, that when the father comes home from work, tired and weary, and mom greets him that the focus of their conversation is often about how the daughter did in school today. When he comes home, there is usually a brief exchange that goes something like this.

Mr. D: God, what a day.
Mrs. D: Yeah, well, it wasn't so easy here either.
Mr. D: More problems with the school?
Mrs. D: They called again. You are going to have to speak to her.
Mr. D: You talk to her. Maybe she'll listen to you.

The worker has noticed that this pattern is common in the family. The couple meets, needing the normal support of one another, and they fall quickly into discussing the daughter, ignoring their own needs for support and nurturing from each other. The daughter provides a safe territory, one where the needs of the individual adults are not exposed. They draw her into their relationship, even when she is not present. In this way, she provides a safety valve for them; she saves them from experiencing themselves.

Over time, as often happens in these situations, one of their children has developed problems. In this case a bright girl is failing in school and is on the edge of being expelled for the year because of her behavior toward teachers and her disruptive behavior in the classroom. The worker has become involved in an attempt to help the parents help their daughter. Both parents express a concern about her behavior and appear to want it to change.

One evening, as the parents and the worker are simply talking together over coffee in the family's home, the worker casually suggests that one of the things that seems to be happening in this family is that the parents seldom seem to discuss themselves with each other. The worker notices that when the subject of their relationship or how they feel toward each other is raised, they end up talking about something else.

Then the worker asks the couple how they are doing together, as a couple. The father replies that they are doing fine together and that if they could just solve this problem with their daughter, they would be able to talk about other things. The mother says that she does not have much time to think about that because she is so worried about what is going to happen with her daughter if she does not get a proper education. She then references her own experience of growing up without an education and says that she is concerned that her daughter will make some of the same mistakes. The father nods his head and says that they have tried everything, but the girl just does not seem to care. The mother interjects that they have met with the schoolteachers, talked with the family doctor, and now are meeting with the worker: "Doesn't that show how concerned we are?

The worker stops the exchange and says, "Let's look at what is happening. I think we are doing just what I was talking about. I ask you how you are doing together, as a couple, and the next thing we know, here we are talking about your daughter. It seems to me that this is just what I was referring to a few minutes ago."

The mother turns to look at her husband, who turns to the worker and, with a laugh, says, "You're right. That's what we do all the time."

This intervention with the family is not going to change things overnight, but it does set the stage for the worker to define this as something they might work on together, especially during those times when the worker is with the family and this dynamic arises. In this case, later that week the worker was in the family home one evening just after dad came home.

The parents and the worker were sitting on the porch talking about what they were going to do about helping each other through this difficult time when the daughter arrived. The father harshly said to her, "You sit right down here, young lady. You and I are going to talk about your attitude at school." Before the exchange had a chance to go any farther, the worker was able to interject.

"Mr. Davids. Before you talk with Darlene, can you and Mrs. Davids and I go for a short walk?"

The father was taken aback, looked at the mother, and they agreed.

As they walked, the child and youth care worker was cautious but clear. "I know that it is important that you talk with Darlene. But for the past few minutes we have been sitting here talking about the two of you. Darlene arrived and all of a sudden it seems like the right time to speak to her. I am remembering the times we have talked about how you struggle to talk with each other, and so end up talking about something else, especially Darlene. Is this one of those times?"

> *Exercise VI: Imagine how the following patterns or dynamics might show up in simple everyday life interactions for a family.*

- One parent defers to the other in terms of decision-making about their youth.
- One parent is able to feel meaningful because the other is always unable to handle situations with the adolescent.
- An adolescent is abusive in interactions with others.
- A child is unable to assert her desires to others.

Interventions Reflect a Way of Connecting Which Fits the Family

Being in relationship, engagement, connectedness: these are characteristics frequently associated with the practice of child and youth care. But how does one become connected or engaged with a family. This section attempts to offer some examples of things a youth care worker might attend to when concerned with connecting with a family in a manner that fits for the family. It is important we note that we are concerned here about connecting with a particular family because, just like all individuals, each family is unique and what counts as a connecting action with one family may not be seen as such by another.

> *Exercise VII: Imagine that when you were an adolescent, your family needed help in dealing with a problem. What are the actions of a helper that would have stimulated your family to reject the helper? What are the actions that would have stimulated the family to accept the helper? What are the reasons why your family would have either wanted to accept or reject the helper?*

The reasons a family may be more or less open to forming a helping relationship with a worker are as varied as families. In considering the exercise above, you may have noticed that your family may have wanted to reject the family because the helper:

- broke a family rule,
- disrespected a family role,
- moved out of sync with your family rhythm, or
- used an inappropriate style.

While there are, of course, other reasons why a family may accept or reject an invitation to engagement, these are the most common. The rest of this section will address these four important concerns.

Rules. All systems have rules. In many cases these rules, as Minuchen (1978) said, are about who can participate and how they can participate in the family. While there are many rules we might expect to be common to most families, as helpers we are most concerned about rules as they are idiosyncratic to the particular family. Within families, some rules are explicit and may be shared with outsiders and even spoken of in the family. For example, the children call all adults over the age of thirty by their family name, money is only given if you work for it, the parents do not discuss family business with the children.

Other rules within families may be implicit. They are not discussed either within the families or with outsiders. These implicit rules are frequently more powerful than the explicit rules because they are secret and not available for discussion or negotiation. For example, in this family we do not discuss sex, we don't talk about dad's drinking, we wait for mother's approval before we discuss things, we never discuss family business with outsiders.

As Ward (1998) has noted, these rules that help to define how one is expected to be in this family can be so embedded that people are just expected to pick them up as they go along. In other words, they are not taught–only learned.

Rules serve a purpose within the family. They may help to maintain an important order within the family, to protect the children or to keep secrets, for example. They help the family maintain the status quo and also help to define who is inside and who is outside the family.

> *Exercise VIII: Describe some of the explicit and implicit rules of your family. What was the purpose of these rules? What happened when they were violated? Were there times when it was acceptable to violate them? Were there people who were allowed to do so?*

Roles. Roles exist in all families, whether it be traditional roles such as parent, brother, sister, or less traditional roles such as scapegoat, savior, or switchboard. These roles serve a purpose: They help the family maintain its structure and manner of interaction. Sometimes they are the corner-posts on which family patterns are anchored. Whatever the reason for their presence, they are fundamental to the functioning of any particular family. Like rules, they may be overt or covert, and they may be played out in a manner idiosyncratic to the family. For example, the role of parent may look very different in different families, depending on the history, traditions, needs, and abilities of the family.

In engaging with families the worker needs to attend to these roles and to how they are manifest within the family. If we fail to pay attention to roles, we may accidentally end up challenging a role that is important for the family to protect, and if we do that, then the family may feel forced to adopt a defensive position towards engagement with us. This is not to suggest that the worker should never challenge the roles in a family; rather, any challenging should be intentional, not accidental.

Imagine, for example, that a father has developed the role of gatekeeper within the family. In order for one to enter into this family system one must go through the father or, in order for information to enter the family system in a meaningful way, it must flow through the father. Why this role exists depends on the particular dynamics of the family. It may be a necessary role to protect family secrets or it may have evolved because of the need, within the family, for the father to feel powerful or for someone else to feel protected.

Now imagine that, as a helper new to this family, you attempt to make contact with the family through the mother. You may find that she fails to discuss matters in depth with you, that she does not call you back, or that she is constantly referring you to the father. This reaction of the mother, which you may want to define as resistance, may in fact simply be a behavior designed to maintain the family structure and functioning. Thus, this behavior to which we are reacting is simply feedback: feedback on the structure of the family, feedback on our approach, or feedback on how we should be with this family. In inviting the mother to become the contact person, we are also inviting her to violate her husband's role in the family. Just as there may be a reaction to our attempts to violate the role, so there may be a consequence for any family member who violates established roles. Our invitation may in fact be an invitation to family disloyalty.

> *Exercise IX: Think of a family that you know. What are the roles that exist in this family. What purpose do these roles serve? What might happen if you were to violate these roles? What are the simple ways in which these roles might be an issue in your working with this family?*

Rhythm and Timing. Child and youth care has for some time been concerned with the idea of rhythmicity in developing connectedness with youth (Desjardins & Freeman, 1991; Kruger, 1991, 2002; Maier, 1994). Like an individual, each family has its own rhythm, and energy seems to come and go. There are times when the family is "up" and times when it is down. We are not talking about the energies of the individuals within the family, although their rhythm and energy does influence the ebb and flow of family energy. We are talking about the sense of energy within the family as a whole. Think of it in general terms for a moment. Imagine a family of two parents, both of whom work, and three children. Now think about a possible weekday.

As the sun rises the house is quiet and calm as family members roll over into the last few minutes of sleep. Twenty minutes later one of the youth is pounding on the bathroom door, demanding his turn at the salon of image creation. In the kitchen, one of the parents is rushing around, a cup of coffee in one hand, putting food on the table. The other parent is rapidly organizing the notes for a meeting while one of the children is asking about plans for the afternoon. Soon everyone is out the door.

Later, at supper, a fight erupts between two of the children, and the parents move to calm it while ensuring that the third is eating sufficiently. After dinner, there is a period of quiet lasting for an hour as the children have retreated to their rooms and one parent sits in front of the television while the other finishes cleaning the kitchen. After this small break, the house again erupts with activity for a few hours. Then as evening falls, people wander off to bed, and the parents sit together in the kitchen with a final cup of tea.

This brief, idealistic overview shows one rhythm of the family, in this case very much influenced by external variables like work and school, activities, and routines. Even in this brief scenario, we can see the possible influences on engagement of the family rhythm. We would not, for example, try to make initial contact during the morning rush or the evening battle. This is not to say we would not be involved in these differing points of routine-driven rhythm. Actually, these may be the very places where we want to work with the family, although perhaps not in the initial stages of connecting. And there are other rhythms of this type in the family. Think now of the rhythm of the week and we can see how it might be different on the weekend than during the week, or the rhythms of the year, influenced by the seasons. In spring, a particular family may be focused on planting and in the fall on harvest and storage as they supplement their food supply. Again, these are externally driven rhythms.

There are other important rhythms within the family. Rhythms of intimacy, for example, which reflects the family's availability to being close with one another or talking about issues of relationship. We may notice that at times the family is more available to one another emotionally, and at other times they are unavailable for such contact. We may notice that at times they express affection and at other times seem distant from one another. We may notice that at times they are open to reflection, and at other times they are not. At times the family may seem to "come together," and at other times they may seem far apart, each member in their own separate world. Sometimes we sense them as a whole, sometimes as scattered parts.

Rhythms like these are particular to the individual family. Energy, openness, availability are important rhythms to watch when working with families, because our ability to connect and engage with a particular family may be influenced by these. If we try to get them all together at a time when they are into a "being distant" mode, we may not meet with success. If we try to discuss intimacy at a time when they are not available for it, we may find our efforts being rejected.

There are other rhythms, of course, in all families. And there are the rhythms inherent in the individual interactions. This section was simply intended to raise this concept as one worthy of attention, not to list all the possibilities. Central to this discussion is, of course, the notion of the timing of our interventions with a particular family. We sometimes think of timing in global terms, as in the time of this family's life, or in more specific terms as in what came just before our intervention. We need also to think of timing in terms of rhythmicity, for the closer we can match ourselves with the rhythm of the family, the more likely we are to be successful in our attempts to create connectedness. If the rhythm is off, the timing cannot be right.

Style. Finally, style is the active manifestation of yourself. It encompasses your language, nonverbal actions, and overall presentation. Ricks (1993) has discussed this in terms of personal position. When we wish to connect with families, we would be wise to consider how we present ourselves, relative to how the family and individual members present themselves. Take, for example, the simple matter of dress. I once knew a worker who went to visit families who lived in poverty. She arrived at their homes in her Mercedes, wearing a fur coat and silk shirts. Her argument for these displays of wealth was that it showed that she was a professional and gave them something to aim for in improving their own lot in life.

Not surprisingly, she had trouble connecting with her clients. It was not only her dress that made a difference. Obviously, there was also the question of attitude. But when she so obviously dressed in a manner that implied, "I am better than you," it surely affected the family's willingness to be relaxed and open with her.

Language too is an issue of immediate concern. If your language is filled with jargon or slang, if the structure of your communications is foreign to the family, or if your words flaunt an education beyond the immediate ability of the family, you may be creating a barrier to engagement in the first encounter.

Finally, there is the issue of overall presentation of self: how you manifest your values, beliefs, ethics, and attitudes in interactions with others. Are you too casual? Too formal? Is there a flow to your way of being with people? Do you present a superior tone or imply judgment in your responses to them? How do others experience you?

> *Exercise X: Enter into a role-playing conversation with three other people in which you are the helper and they are a family you are trying to help. Discuss an issue of concern to the family and try to be helpful. After 10 minutes stop the role play and ask each of them to give you some feedback on how they experienced you.*

In this section I have been concerned with some of the issues involved in developing ways of connecting that fit the families with a special focus on en-

gagement. Throughout your work with families and well beyond the early stages
of engagement, you will need to be concerned with creating interventions that
fit for the particular family. This focus on early connections is simply a way to
highlight the importance of this issue of fit.

It is not, of course, that we must only be concerned with how we fit in terms
of roles, rules, rhythm, and style. Our interventions must also fit with the family in many other ways. While it is not possible here to address fully the issues
involved in creating interventions that fit, some of the other areas of concern
include:

1. Does your intervention fit with the family's conceptualization of their
   problem? If it does not fit for them, they may not respond as you might
   hope.
2. Is your intervention appropriate to the developmental stage of the family?
3. Does your immediate intervention fit with the overall direction with the
   family?
4. Does your intervention fit with the cultural aspects of the family?
5. Is your intervention congruent with the family way of operating in the
   world?

Throughout our work with families, we are constantly asking ourselves,
"Does what I am about to do fit this family?" If we fail to ask this question, we
run the risk of developing standardized responses across differing family situations. For a further discussion of the idea of "interventions that fit" see Garfat
(1998). We turn now to the process of intervention.

A BRIEF FRAMEWORK FOR CHILD AND YOUTH CARE

Interventions with Families

In order to be effective in working with youth or families, child and youth
care workers need a framework for understanding the process of intervention,
for it is this framework that helps the worker decide what to do next at each
stage of the process (Ricks & Garfat, 1989). Historically, while we have focused on strategies and interventions, we have done so in the absence of such
an organizing framework (see Garfat & Newcomen, 1992). It is the intention
of this section to provide such a framework. This framework, which involves
the processes of *Noticing, Reflection, Preparation, and Intervention*, will not
help the worker in terms of the content of interventions, only in terms of the
process. As mentioned previously, the content of our interventions are very
much determined by the theoretical frame or lens which each of us uses, and
such a lens is developed out of a combination of one's values, beliefs and ethics.

The framework presented here evolved from my experience in working with child and youth care workers over the years and is, in fact, a reflection of the process that seems to be associated with effective child and youth care interventions (Garfat, 1998).

Noticing

The process of intervention begins with noticing: noticing what is going on "out there" in the world of interactions and noticing what is going on "in here" in the personal world of experiencing of the worker. The two, however, are intricately related, because what one notices out there is very much influenced by the inner world of the child and youth care worker. For example, if one believes that change occurs because of external events, one may tend to notice things such as how people reinforce one another. On the other hand, if one believes that change occurs because of a shift in how people make meaning of a situation, one may look for evidence of how people are interpreting their experiences and responding to that interpretation.

The inner world of the worker is something that, regardless of the theoretical framework one adopts, must be a part of the noticing in the early stages of intervention. As well as "seeing how one is seeing," the worker must also notice the internal experiences she is having. For example, one may see the action of the mother in the opening of this chapter as appropriate or inappropriate and, depending on how one defines her actions, one may be attracted to it, repelled by it, frightened, shocked, or experience any other range of emotions in response to it. If one fails to notice how one is responding personally to the actions and experiences "out there," one runs the risk of reacting to the situation from a personal bias rather than proactively responding according to the needs of the family at the moment.

We also notice the opportunity for intervention. A situation arises, or is created, within which the child and youth care worker sees the opportunity to take an action intentionally directed to impact the family, either through impacting an individual, a subgroup, or in the ways that individuals are in interaction with one another.

In summary, then, we have a situation where the worker experiences a situation, gives meaning to it, and responds to that meaning by interpreting it as an opportunity for intervention. Internal experiencing on a personal level may taint the workers response, just as a more objective professional frame might influence it. So it is not so much what you see out there that is important in the noticing as it is what you do with what you see.

Exercise XI: Join with a colleague or friend to watch a group of at least three people interact. Watch them for about five minutes. When you stop watching, discuss with your colleague the following:

What did you each notice "out there?" What did you actually see–not your interpretation of it but what did you actually witness? How were your "noticings" the same? Were there things you both observed? How were your "noticings" different? What did one of you notice that the other did not?

Now discuss the things you both saw and how each of you interpreted these. You will have discovered that either you noticed different things or that you noticed the same things and some of them you interpreted differently? Why do you suppose that is? How is it that you have come to notice the things you do and to interpret them in the manner that you do?

As you observe them, identify opportunities for intervention. What makes these opportunities for you? Do your colleagues see different opportunities? Discuss these. What would you have to do in order to agree with your colleagues that these are opportunities? What does that say about you?

Reflecting

Once one has noticed either what is going on out there or what is going on in here and interpreted it as an opportunity for intervention, it is useful to take a little time to reflect on what one sees or what is going on. This is, perhaps, as much as anything else a central and necessary part of the process of creating interventions that fit for the family and for the current situation. In an inquiry into the elements associated with effective child and youth care interventions Garfat (1998) identified a number of elements of context which seem important in creating such interventions. The following describes some of these elements and adapts them in consideration of the context of interventions with families.

It is important to remember as one reads through the following that each element applies to all of the persons who are a party to the intervention. Thus in the example given at the beginning, each element applies equally to the mother, the father, each of the youth and, importantly, to the child and youth care worker. Each of these elements impacts on our choice of intervention, which will be discussed in the following section. The worker is essentially involved in the process of giving meaning to his or her experiencing (Bruner, 1990).

History of caregiving and care-receiving. Each of us has a unique history of caring experiences and experiencing that impact how we might experience and respond to any given event in the present. In the case of the family intervention, it would appear that our previous experiences of being the receiver of caring actions, whether professional or personal, help to define what counts as caring for us. Thus, for example, pointing something out to me may be something that I associate as caring because of how I have experienced it in the past. Similarly, I may interpret pointing something out as threatening because of experiences in my past in which I was hurt or punished after someone pointed something out to me. We need, therefore, to know some of what counts as caring for each member of the family and for ourselves.

In this simple example, we see the complexity of the family intervention because, while a particular intervention may count as caring for one member of the family, it may be experienced differently by another because of an individual history. Thus in making a decision about which intervention to use, the worker must consider the possible impact of the intervention on each of the members of the family.

Personal position. Everyone has what Ricks (1993) has called a personal position or a particular presentation of self and an orientation to the world based on their own values, beliefs, and ethics. This is of particular importance for the worker, because this personal position will directly impact on how the worker is experiencing and valuing their experience with the family. We all have a tendency to think that the way we see the world is the way the world is (Watzlawick, 1990). The way that we view the world shows up in our personal position. The more we become aware of our personal position, the less likely we are to choose an intervention just because we think it is right rather than because it is of particular relevance for this family at this time.

Family history. Each person has a unique family history, even if raised in the same family. Within each family there exists what Bruner (1990) has called a folk psychology, a particular way of seeing the world and giving meaning to particular events. We learn this folk psychology in our family of origin and we carry it with us into the families we develop. This is one of the reasons why couples sometimes have conflicts about how to raise or parent their children. Each may value different approaches. Also, within our new families we develop certain of our ways of responding to individual actions; we develop a new family folk psychology based on the experiences we have together. Being aware of the family folk psychology helps us to structure our interventions in a manner that fits for the family.

Culture. Like family experiences, the culture of our origin and the culture in which we live have a great impact on how we act and understand. Knowing and understanding the culture of the families with whom we work is essential if we are to avoid making careless errors that distance us from the family members. For example, it is easy for a person to misinterpret a worker's intention if the manner of expressing that intention has a different interpretation within the other culture.

Other items of context. It is not possible here to discuss all the elements of context that might be associated with the effectiveness of our interventions. Some of these include the participants' experiences of time and timing, space, the organizational atmosphere which defines acceptable and unacceptable interventions, as well as our own anxieties, fears, and personal passions. The reader interested in other elements of context that impact the intervention and are therefore relevant to our reflection during the process of intervention are directed to Garfat (1998).

Relationships are central to child and youth care work in all its various forms. In working with families we need to attend to the quality and characteristics of the relationships we have with each member of the family and with the family as a whole. Because of our own history as child and youth care workers we may have an unfortunate tendency to value or focus on our relationship with the identified youth to the detriment of the other relationships we have with family members. We must attend to the quality and characteristics of the relationships between family members and between family members and other important persons in the life of the family.

> *Exercise XII: Join with a group of colleagues in observing a family in interaction. It is not important that the family is having a problem at the time of your observations. As you watch the family, identify what elements of context, as suggested above, seem to be influencing the interaction. Discuss these with your colleagues. Identify why the particular elements of context that you have identified (which may also be different than those identified above) are important to you. How did you come to value these?*

Notice that you are making meaning here. What is the implication of how you make meaning for your work with families?

Preparation

Once we have recognized an opportunity for intervention and taken the time to consider the aspects of context that might be relevant to the current situation, we need to take a little more time to prepare for the actual intervention. This may sound like we are taking a lot of time here but, in reality, once the process becomes habit for the child and youth care worker, this process occurs almost instantly on a subconscious level. The following, in no particular order, are some of the areas we might consider in preparing for actual intervention.

Considering alternative interventions. Part of preparing for intervention is deciding which of many interventions to use. In any given situation there is always more than one possibility available for the worker. In order to make a decision about which intervention to use, the worker must take the time to actually think about what options are available. In simple terms this requires the worker

to brainstorm alternatives. Too often the worker simply uses the first intervention that comes to mind when that may not necessarily be the intervention of
choice. In considering which intervention to use, the worker considers things such
as:

1. How might this intervention be interpreted by different family members?
2. What might be their reactions?
3. Is it developmentally appropriate?
4. Is the worker capable of doing the intervention?
5. Can it be completed within the time available?
6. How does it fit into the overall understanding of, and direction for, the
   family?

Preparation of self. Child and youth care work involves the use of self in relationship, because child and youth care is a relationship-based form of intervention. Thus, in making preparation for intervention it is essential that the
child and youth care worker "check in with self." What this particular expression means will depend on your interpretation of the word "self" and which aspects
of self are important to you. Minimally, the worker must note

a. the current state of the worker's emotional self,
b. the personal position one has adopted vis-à-vis the current situation,
c. the meaning one is making of the current situation, and
d. the worker's current state of availability for connection with others.

Checking in with self actually refers to the workers' personal readiness to
carry out the intervention or, in other words, asking, "How am I doing here?" In
checking with self, for example, the worker may notice that she is currently
frightened for her physical safety or disconnected with the current interactions.
The worker may discover that there is something she needs to do in order to be
ready to intervene in a manner that is focused on the family or family member.
Obviously, this must be attended to before the worker can proceed.

Connection and availability. In order for an intervention to be effective the
family, or family members, towards whom the intervention is directed must be
ready (available) to receive the intervention. Being ready in this context refers
to the idea that the person towards whom the intervention is directed must minimally be in connection with the worker, must be focused on the current interaction, and must be emotionally or cognitively capable, at the current moment,
to receive the intervention being considered. The worker will experience self
as being present and in relationship with the family members to whom the intervention is directed when this connectedness exists. A potentially great intervention can be rendered meaningless if the family member is, for example, too

distracted by other thoughts to attend to the worker or if the worker is not connected in relationship.

Referencing theory or knowledge. Every effective child and youth care worker is a repository of knowledge that may have come from their studies, their work, or their personal life experience. Through these we learn about groups, families, and individuals. Thus, part of preparation for intervention involves the process of accessing the knowledge of the worker about the current family and situation. For example, a family may be struggling with setting limits for a young adolescent, and the worker may notice that this is the family's first adolescent, thus marking a particular stage of family development. Or in a blended family the worker may notice that one parent has taken a role in parenting that excludes the other, and the worker may have had previous experience in working with blended families from which she has gained certain knowledge about negotiating parenting roles. In any given situation, therefore, the worker must ask, "What knowledge do I have (or need) that may have relevance in this situation?"

Preparing to take responsibility. Effective child and youth care workers are prepared to take responsibility for whatever comes of their actions or interventions. By this it is not meant that the worker is prepared to accept blame but, rather, that they recognize that their actions will have consequences and they are prepared to deal with whatever the outcome may be. For example, if a worker joins with a father in chopping wood, the worker will be prepared to follow-up on whatever comes in response. The worker has an intention that everything will work out and takes responsibility for trying to ensure that happens. The responsible worker does not blame the family members for a lack of progress but, rather, looks seriously at her role in any lack of progress, without blaming herself either.

> *Exercise XIII: Observe, with your colleagues, a family group in interaction. As before, identify opportunities and reflect on the relevant elements of context and how you make meaning of what you are seeing. Now, thinking about the opportunity you have observed, identify a number of interventions that might be possible at this point. Consider each of the interventions in terms of how they might be interpreted by individual family members and each person's possible reaction to them. Consider each, as well, in terms of how it might be related to the overall goals with this family. Discuss how you would feel about making each of the interventions. Identify the one that feels right, and why.*

Intervention

The final phase involves the actual act of intervening. Within this phase the worker might be concerned with three specific tasks: connecting, attending to feedback, and the action of intervening.

As mentioned, for an intervention to be effective, the worker must be in a connected relationship with the family member(s) to whom the intervention is directed. Thus, as the first step of actually delivering the intervention, the worker makes a final check to insure that the individual is focused on the worker enough to attend to the intervention. In simple terms this may mean that the worker has to make contact with an individual or, in more complex terms, it may mean that the worker needs to draw the attention of the whole family group to the current process.

At all stages of working with the family and, especially, as the worker goes through the process of intervention, feedback is available for interpretation. Attending to this feedback helps the worker to notice the family members' response to her actions and provides information which may suggest, for example, that a modification to the intervention process is necessary. Imagine for a moment that a worker has asked a parent to join the worker and the youth on a walk. As the worker makes the request, the other parent may move away from the parent who has been asked. This action represents feedback, which must be interpreted in terms of what the worker knows about this family in particular and human behavior in general. It may signal, for example, that this is dangerous territory or that this is a typical pattern of disengagement from potentially stressful parenting situations or that there is a lack of support for the actions of the worker. Depending, therefore, on how the worker interprets this action, she may decide to withdraw from the intervention or to modify the style of the intervention or to change her own physical location during the intervention.

When the intervention is actually undertaken, it is done so with the intention that it will be effective, with the best interests of all family members in the forefront and in a manner that respects the personal integrity of the individual family members. The worker's belief in the intervention would seem to be an important element in whether or not the intervention is going to be successful. Finally, interventions that are related to the immediate process and connected to the overall process of work with the family are those which have the greatest impact (Garfat, 1998). Thus, for example, in the case where one parent has withdrawn from the majority of parenting responsibility in difficult situations, and when the greater involvement of this parent in those situations has been identified as a goal of working with the family, then an intervention which is addressed to this dynamic, as it is occurring, would likely be more impactful than an intervention directed to the pattern when it is not occurring. Such an intervention would, of course, also be consistent with the child and youth care approach of intervening into daily life situations as they are occurring.

Exercise XIV: Enter into a role-play situation with a family whose difficulty is characteristic of the families with whom you normally expect to work.

Have this role-play occur in the family's living space, not an office workspace. Let the family's natural patterns of interacting occur, let them live their life with you in their presence, just as the family did in the example which opened this article. Ask a group of colleagues to observe the situation.

After the role-play has evolved for a few minutes, stop and discuss with your colleagues whatever you are noticing, "out there" and "in here." Find out from them what other things they are noticing. Re-enter the role-play and continue with it until you notice an opportunity for intervention.

Stop the role-play again and reflect on this opportunity with your colleagues. Allow them to help you understand how you are giving meaning to what you are experiencing. Discuss possible interventions and how the individual family members might respond to them. Choose an intervention and engage in the process of preparation.

Re-enter the role again and make the intervention. Stop the role-play.

Discuss with the family members their experience of you, how they interpreted the intervention, their speculations about how you could have been more effective, and their overall experience of you as a child and youth care worker in this situation.

The foregoing describes a simple process of intervention that a child and youth care worker might follow in working with families. In outlining this process I have also tried to indicate some of the things that a worker might want to consider along the way. In order to close, we now return to the scenario described at the beginning. Before reading further, please re-read that description and the questions that followed it.

CONCLUSION: ANSWERING THE QUESTIONS

In this final section, I offer some possible answers to the questions posed at the beginning. It is important to understand that this is simply one worker's response to a situation based on who he is and how he interprets what he experiences with this family at this time, given how he knows them. With another worker or another family, in a similar situation, or with a different orientation, the worker's responses may have been different—and equally valid.

Why are they in the house rather than an office? And why the kitchen?

This worker is a child and youth care worker committed to the values that underlay a child and youth care approach to families. Thus, he would rather be with the family where their life is lived so he can experience it as it unfolds rather than hear it described. Further, he believes that if he can help them change their patterns of interacting in the environment in which that interacting occurs, any changes are more likely to be integrated into their patterns of living.

They are in the kitchen because this is a rural environment where sitting around the kitchen is the natural culture. As well, given the limited space in this family home, tasks like fly-tying tend to occur at the kitchen table. Metaphorically, the kitchen table is the center of the home and family life.

Why are the worker, father, and son talking about fly fishing as opposed to, for example, talking about the youth's difficulties in school or with his parents?

Based on his experience of this family so far, the worker believes that it would be valuable for the father and the son to be involved in some common, relatively normal, father-son type activities. This is a goal that the family has been able to accept at this stage as something that they think would improve family life. It is also the worker's hope that if the father and son can begin to do some non-stressful, enjoyable activities together, the father may become more involved in other aspects of the son's life from which he has withdrawn. In this cultural environment, with this family, fishing is something they might do together, and it is something at which the father has a special skill, so he is able to assume the role of teacher or guide with his son, thereby defining part of his role as such.

The parents have spent a lot of time over the past few years with other professionals talking about the son's difficulties in school and with his parents. So much so, in fact, that talking about these problems has become a recognizable pattern within the family. Together, they are hoping to develop some new patterns of interaction based on positive experiences together. The father and son are doing this together without the mother or the other children, because the father and son need to learn again how to be together in these particular roles. Part of the worker's job here is actually to keep the other family members out of this action, thereby helping the family to learn a little about appropriate boundaries, another area in which they struggle.

What is the meaning of the mother being asleep while the worker, the dad, and the youth are talking?

What something means depends, as we have seen, on a number of factors. Based on the worker's experience of the family, and some direct questions, the worker knows something of how mom's daytime naps, discussed briefly on a previous visit, are interpreted. In this case, for the father, it means that his wife is still sick and depressed. They have both been sick a lot over the past few years, and he seems to think that this is an indication of how difficult life is. The mother says that her sleeping represents a tiredness that comes from how much energy she puts into the difficulties caused by Bobby. Bobby, on the other hand, sees her sleeping as an indication of what a problem he is and how much she does not really like him because of that. The other two children, in the living room, think that mom has to sleep a lot because Bobby's problems have made her sick. We see then that with the exception of the father, the family is in agreement that mom's sleeping is an outcome of Bobby's disturbance. The worker has a hypothesis that it is a way in which the mother forces the father to be involved to some degree with the children.

How is it that mom's volume, intensity, and style do not change when she sees the worker sitting in the kitchen?

It is important to understand that the mother does not see any problem with her manner of interacting with the children or her husband. Why should she change a behavior that, for her, is not problematic? Further, her explosive reaction makes a statement to the worker about how hard her life is and how the father does not involve himself. Of course, we also notice that her reaction serves as a focal point for engagement with the father. This is a typical pattern in this family, whereby the children serve as a focus of conversation and interaction between the parents.

The worker has seen this same pattern before and has also noticed that, as the children's volume increases, the father does nothing to prevent it. Indeed, it has seemed to the worker at times that the father is waiting for the mother to come out of the room. Yelling at the father also seems to be an outlet for her other frustrations in her relationship with him.

Why is the worker not intervening with the siblings?

The worker could have intervened directly with the siblings to calm them, or he could have asked the father to intervene and supported him in doing so, but he chose not to do so. Part of the worker's struggle has also to do with his awareness that he needs to help the family define appropriate boundaries, and he is unsure if dealing with the other children will encourage them to continue to interrupt the father-son relationship as it is changing. The truth is that the worker was afraid to intervene directly with the youth himself. He was concerned about how it would look to the father if he intervened and was not successful. He tells himself that he did not want to interrupt this moment with the father and son in order to suggest that the father intervene himself.

The worker rationalizes his behavior by telling himself that soon the mother would come out of her room annoyed, and that is what he really wanted to deal with. The result of the worker's decision is that he might have missed a wonderful opportunity to help the father become more involved with parenting all the children. The worker obviously has some work of his own to do.

Why did the worker not ask for the mother to join him?

When mom came out of the room, the worker was caught off-guard and was not sure what to do. Rather than asking her to join them at the table, he chose to let the situation play itself out a little while he gathered his thoughts and presence. He had seen this before and was not worried about any harm, but he also knew that he had to respond–and be seen to respond–in some manner. Later, when he and the parents are talking about the situation, they identify that this is something specific that they will work on together so that the next time the worker notices the father not involving himself with the other youth, he can reference this discussion. It marked an important point in redefining the problem as not just about Bobby but about the family functioning.

Unsure about what to do, the worker was about to jump in when he remembered a few things: "If you deal with a pattern when it is highly emotional you are less likely to be successful and, if you intervene too quickly, you might not discover the purpose of the behavior." By letting it go this time the worker was able to confirm his thinking that the behavior served to engage the parents with each other. The father needed this behavior as much as the mother.

Does it matter that it is spring?

In this case, it does. This is a poor family and they are dependent on their own resources to supplement their basic needs for food. In the spring they plant a large garden which they tend throughout the summer and harvest in the fall. Fishing also supplements their diet. During the winter the father gathers squirrel tails, feathers, and other natural things to make fishing lures. The ritual of fly-tying marks a transition from a more difficult time (winter) to an easier time (summer) and is therefore a symbol of the natural rhythm of this family. By being involved in this manner the worker is connecting himself with this rhythm. Further, if the son gets involved in the fly-tying and fishing ritual with the father, he will be more involved in the family life in an important and contributing way.

What should the worker do at this point?

This question brings us to the final exercise in this chapter and represents a final opportunity for you to apply your own orientation to this situation.

Exercise XV: It is time for an intervention, and it is your responsibility to intervene. Reflecting on what has been said so far, identify what you think the worker should do at this point in the scenario.

It has been the intention of this chapter to assist the reader in developing a child and youth care orientation toward working with families. We have reviewed some of the assumptions that underlay such an approach, identified some of the characteristics that may be associated with effective child and youth care interventions with families, and looked at a brief overview of the process of intervention.

Child and youth care work with families is a complicated process involving all of the workers skills. It differs from other forms of intervention and is particular to the field. It represents an exciting new challenge for workers who have previously been involved only with youth, and it expands the opportunities for us to be helpful.

REFERENCES

Austin, D., & Halpin, W. (1989). The caring response. *Journal of Child and Youth Care, 4*(3), 1-7.

Bruner, J. (1990). *Acts of meaning*. Cambridge, MA: Harvard University Press.

Dejardins, S., & Freeman, A. (1991). Out of synch. *Journal of Child and Youth Care, 6*(4), 139-144.

Fewster, G. (1990). *Being in child care: A journey into self*. New York: The Haworth Press, Inc.

Fox, L. (1995). Exploiting daily events to heal the pain of sexual abuse. *Journal of Child and Youth Care, 10*(2), 33-42.

Garfat, T. (1992). Reflections on the journal entries of a residential hunter. *Journal of Child and Youth Care, 7*(3), 59-66.

Garfat, T. (1994). Never alone: Reflections on the presence of self and history on child and youth care. *Journal of Child and Youth Care Work, 9*(1), 35-43.

Garfat, T. (1998). Developing effective child and youth care interventions. *Journal of Child and Youth Care, 12*(1/2), 1-178.

Garfat T., & Newcomen, T. (1992). AS*IF: A model for child and youth care interventions. *Child and Youth Care Forum 21*(4), 277-285.

Josselson, R. (1992). *The space between us: Exploring the dimensions of human relationships*. San Francisco: Jossey-Bass.

Krueger, M. A. (1991). Coming from your center, being there, meeting them where they're at, interacting together, counselling on the go, creating circles of caring, discovering and using self, and caring for one another: Central themes in professional child and youth care. *Journal of Child and Youth Care, 5*(1), 77-87.

Krueger, M. (1994). Rhythm and presence: Connecting with children on the edge. *Journal of Emotional and Behavioral Problems, 3*(1), 49-51.

Krueger, M. (1998). *Interactive youth work practice*. Washington, DC: Child Welfare League of America.

Krueger, M. (in press). *In the rhythms of youth: Themes and stories in youth work practice*. New York: The Haworth Press, Inc.

Maier, H. W. (1979). The core of care: Essential ingredients for the development of children at home and away from home. *Child Care Quarterly 8*(3), 161-173.

Maier, H. W. (1987). *Developmental group care for children and youth: Concepts and practice*. New York: The Haworth Press, Inc.

Maier, H. W. (1992). Rhythmicity–A powerful force for experiencing unity and personal connections. *Journal of Child and Youth Care Work, 5*, 7-13.

Minuchen, S. (1978). *Families and family therapy*. Boston: Harvard University Press.

Peterson, R. (1988). The collaborative metaphor technique: Using Ericsonian (Milton H.) techniques and principles in child, family and youth care work. *Journal of Child Care, 3*(4), 11-27.

Redl, F. (1959). Strategy and technique of the life-space interview. *American Journal of Orthopsychiatry, 29*,1-18.

Ricks, F. (1989). Self-awareness model for training and application in child and youth care. *Journal of Child and Youth Care, 4*(1), 33-42.

Ricks, F. (1992). A feminist's view of caring. *Journal of Child and Youth Care, 7*(2), 49-58.

Ricks, F. (1993). Therapeutic education: Personal growth experiences for child and youth care workers. *Journal of Child and Youth Care, 8*(3), 17-34.

Ricks, F., & Garfat, T. (1989). Working with individuals and their families: Considerations for child and youth care workers. *Journal of Child and Youth Care Work, 5*(1), 63-70.

Ward, A. (1998). The inner world and its implications. In A. Ward & L. McMahon (Eds.), *Intuition is not enough*. London: Routledge.

Watzlawick, P. (1990). *Munchhausen's pigtale: Or psychotherapy and reality*. New York: W. W. Norton.

From Front Line to Family Home:
A Youth Care Approach
to Working with Families

Kelly Shaw
Thom Garfat

SUMMARY. This chapter explores the shifts that occur when child and youth care workers begin to move from the relative safety of the residential program into the community to support families to live together more successfully in their own homes. When families are struggling to live together, in-home family intervention, grounded in a child and youth care approach and practiced from within a youth care framework, is a viable intervention option. *[Article copies available for a fee from The Haworth Document Delivery Service: 1-800-HAWORTH. E-mail address: <docdelivery@ haworthpress.com> Website: <http://www.HaworthPress.com> © 2003 by The Haworth Press, Inc. All rights reserved.]*

KEYWORDS. Youthwork with families, youth care work, social work with families, family-centered residential care, child and youth care, family services, family support, parent education, residential care work and families

My career began as a child and youth care (CYC) worker in a program with a mandate to assess youngsters. Youngsters lived in the program for six weeks

---

Kelly Shaw is affiliated with Nexus, Nova Scotia. Thom Garfat is affiliated with TransformAction Consulting & Training, Montreal, Quebec, and is Co-editor of *CYC-Net* (www.cyc-net.org) and *Relational Child and Youth Care Practice*.

[Haworth co-indexing entry note]: "From Front Line to Family Home: A Youth Care Approach to Working with Families." Shaw, Kelly, and Thom Garfat. Co-published simultaneously in *Child & Youth Services* (The Haworth Press, Inc.) Vol. 25, No. 1/2, 2003, pp. 39-53; and: *A Child and Youth Care Approach to Working with Families* (ed: Thom Garfat) The Haworth Press, Inc., 2003, pp. 39-53. Single or multiple copies of this article are available for a fee from The Haworth Document Delivery Service [1-800-HAWORTH, 9:00 a.m. - 5:00 p.m. (EST). E-mail address: docdelivery@haworthpress.com].

while being subject to psychological, educational, and behavioral assessments. A few years later, a decision was made to change the mandate of our program from short-term assessment to long-term treatment, and the program would have a family focus. Outreach and preventative work within the community would also be one of the program's prime objectives.

This change required a change in values as well as goals. When I began working in residential care, parents and families were seen as the cause of the troubled children with whom we worked (Fewster & Garfat, 1993; Garfat & McElwee, 2001). Residential programs and child welfare systems positioned themselves on the child's side, often against the parents (Fewster & Garfat, 1993). There was a sense that we were protecting the child from the family. Often children triangulated the staff with their parents, and while their relationships with adults and community were often more effective while living in residential care, this did not always transfer into the families way of being in relationship or of living together.

I remember late night conversations early in my career talking about "the parents." In these discussions they became horrible creatures. Reflecting back, I am appalled that I participated in such a slanderous activity. However, I began working in residential care when parents delivered their children to treatment to be fixed and then returned to them. Thankfully, I did eventually identify that this was not working. The question is, why not?

Several years later, we began to have conversations about the parents that took a very different direction. No longer slanderous, these conversations focused on solutions. "How can we work differently with the children and youngsters who enter our program?" we asked, because we did not seem to be having much success with our present approach. As a team we began to identify the characteristics of more successful residential treatment for troubled youngsters and children. There also seemed to be problems with the time spent in our residential program and the parental involvement in the treatment process. This realization felt like an illumination. The question then was what we should do?

EXAMINING VALUES AND BELIEFS

In the early days, parents dropped off their children and might call a few times during their youngster's stay. Children did not see their parents during the time that they spent in the program. Parents were not a part of the process. So how does a residential care program make the shift to include parents differently? How can we work with parents and families, not only with the youth?

We found that the first step is to examine what you—as an individual and as a program—believe about families. It is key to explore these beliefs through some personal questions and time for reflection. Some of these questions are: Do you believe parents are the root of all evil? Are the issues of the children simply the issues of the child? Do parents have rights and responsibilities when their child enters residential care? What about siblings? Grandparents? Extended family? What is your definition of family?

As you begin to think about leaving the relative safety of the residential program and move toward working with families, examine why you want to work with families in this way. Personal values about parents and families may include pieces of how you were raised or how you are raising your own children. The program values (e.g., values around violence, views of women and minorities) and the things that we value about our own ways of doing things may not fit the families with whom we are working.

How will you feel when working with a father who has been sexually inappropriate with his son or daughter? What will it mean for you to work with a family while they are blending children from previous marriages? How will you cope with going to the funeral for the favorite grandmother of a youngster with whom you are working? Knowing ourselves is essential to working effectively with youngsters and families (Ricks, 1989). Understanding our prejudices, biases, stereotypes, fears, phobias, needs, and strengths is important so that we can be real with ourselves, our colleagues, and those with whom we work.

Once you begin to explore these issues, you will be confronted with the logistics of how to work with families within a residential framework and how front-line youth care workers make the shift to working with families.

FROM YOUTH TO FAMILY: FROM RESIDENTIAL TO COMMUNITY INTERVENTION

Think about the following activities which any child and youth care worker may engage in with the children with whom they work:

- playing catch
- reading a story
- cooking supper
- doing laundry
- watching a movie
- playing chess
- transitioning towards bedtime

- painting a bedroom
- registering for school
- doing homework

Now imagine what it would be like for a CYC worker to do these activities with children while they are at home with their families. Would the activities change? Would you still do them? Would you do them differently? Would it matter if the parents were there? How? Why?

Working with children, youth and their families, whether in a residential setting or while they are in the community, poses unique challenges. When children are staying in a residential living environment, child and youth care workers will have a different role than they did when parents and families were not included. For example, decisions about how much time the youngster will stay within the residential program will be made with the needs and wants of the family in mind. These decisions will no longer be made arbitrarily by treatment teams or social workers. Parents become partnered in the process of helping their children and family (Whittaker, 1979).

These are shifts that occur as you work with a family over time. Based on your initial assessment, you may be there during their intimate moments, when they are struggling with their children, when they are nestling children into bed, and when they are welcoming them home from school. These experiences change your relationship with and within the family. You do not become a part of the family system, although you become a part of the changes within the family system. Simply by being there, you influence the behaviors and choices that will be made by the people present.

In the early stages of involvement with families in their home, the family may consider you to be company. You may be offered coffee or a beverage. Snacks are made for your arrival, and a special dinner may be prepared because you are going to be there for supper. This has an influence on the family system, and they will be different because you are there. In order to be effective, you must pay attention to the nuances and the rhythm of the family. When are you no longer company? When do you make your own cup of tea? When do you become involved in cooking supper? And how?

When a residential care program begins to work with families, the children in the program are understood in context more than they were before you worked with their family (Kwantes, 1992). Behaviors have a different meaning when you have the family context.

I once worked with a young fellow who had a very foul mouth. I do not mean that he swore in anger or frustration. He swore in general conversation. At the supper table he would ask you to "pass the fuckin' butter, please." Once I spent time in the family home, eating supper with them, I had a different understanding of his behavior. It was part of his family culture. Sitting at the family dinner table hearing the father and siblings all ask politely for condiments using the "f" word made the interpretation of young Sam's language less pathological. It was part of the language of belonging. Later, we were able to shift our focus with this youngster and his parents to talk about when and where you can swear rather than dissect this young lad for the root of the problem.

This story explains something about what we understand CYC work to be. CYC workers like being with young people and not being therapists. It is really not important why a behavior is occurring. It is obviously serving some purpose (Garfat, 2003). It may serve the purpose of helping the young person to belong, as in the foregoing example, or the purpose of helping him feel in control or even simply to feel valuable or of worth. If we can figure out the purpose being served by the behavior, and help the young person to find another way to meet this purpose with another more socially acceptable behavior that is less stressful and/or painful for the youngster and those people who are living with him/her, then this is better.

BEING WHERE THEY LIVE THEIR LIVES

What does it look like to work with a family using a youth care approach? Simply put, it means being with them while they are doing what they do. It means the utilization of daily life events as they are occurring for therapeutic purposes (Garfat, 1995, 1998). It means folding laundry, weeding the garden, tucking children into bed, peeling potatoes, fights about curfew. It means being with families and struggling with them as they change and learn more effective ways of being in relationship with each other.

These are the details that make family work the child and youth care way unique. When we are being therapeutic with a family, just as when we are being this way with a child, we are using daily life events, and sometimes the goals of our interventions are subtle. We are in relationship with individual family members in such a way that it encourages others in the family to be different in relationship with each other. We are intimately a part of the therapeutic process.

INCORPORATING FAMILY VALUES

When you first start to think about working with families, you will have been using treatment or program plans that were developed for individual children. When families become involved, the individual plans need to have a family focus. These plans need to reflect the values and beliefs of individual families. If you want to work with families you have to shift your thinking to include families on a daily basis. You can no longer ask, "Should we let Julie go to the mall Friday after school with her friends?" Instead, you ask, "Would Julie's parents let her go to the mall Friday after school with her friends?" Then you encourage and support Julie to call her parents and ask if she can go to the mall.

I remember a time when 14-year-old James came back to the center with a permission slip to participate in a sexuality education workshop at school. He asked me to sign it. I read that the paper explained the program and asked for parental permission in order for the student to participate. I suggested to James that he call his parents and get their permission over the phone before I would sign it. This evoked a conversation with James about his parents' moral values about sex. He explained that he was uncomfortable calling them. We practiced the call and, after much coaxing, he did call them. His father answered the phone and told James that he thought it was a great opportunity. I then signed the permission slip.

If Julie's parents want her to participate in an activity that the residential program feels is not safe for Julie or conflicts with the treatment plan for the youngster and family, then you are confronted with a teachable moment. For example, if Julie was 12 and her mother thought it would be great to get her belly button pierced for a grading present, and one of the goals that has been identified for Julie is to help her be a young girl, then piercing her belly button would be in conflict with this goal. Mom would be aware of this goal and will need to be supported in parenting Julie to stay a young girl and not to try to grow up too fast. Your relationship with Mom will be invaluable during this engagement. Individual programs take on different meaning when they are written from within the context of family.

We also need to understand that families need support during times of transition. This would include any time when there are changes within the family structure: when a couple begins a family, when infant children become toddlers, when children become adolescents, when adolescent children become adults, when adult children leave home, when a parent dies, when a grand parent dies, when there is job loss or a significant geographical move.

Those of us who work in residential care are familiar with some of these transition stages. However, when working with families who say that they are struggling with their adolescent children, it is remarkable to discover that there are other transition factors present. This may be the death of a parent's parent (a grandparent), the addition of a family member, perhaps a new baby or an older child returning home. An understanding of these developmental stages is an important part of the training a youth care worker should receive before moving towards working with families.

Rules and Roles

As much as child and youth care workers try, they sometimes fall into a parental role with children, especially those living in a residential care program. When a program shifts to working with families, this should happen less. To help you avoid this "parentification," perhaps a change in language would be helpful. Thinking about youngsters as visitors to the residential program rather than residents will keep the parents' involvement and role in the forefront. Children live with their families and stay in the residential unit for a period of time. Ideally they spend regular time at home during the week or perhaps weekends and holidays or maybe they live at home more than they stay at the residential program.

Working with families also means understanding their rules. It is the rules and boundaries that tie families together (Minuchin, 1974). They are the structural frameworks that keep the elements together in a cohesive, organized fashion. These rules, which are a part of all families, may be implicit or explicit. For example, if a family has a socially unacceptable rule, like bigotry, it may not be discussed. This may be relevant when the teenage son begins dating a young woman who is not from the same ethnic background as them. Perhaps this is where the family began having struggles. Families maintain these rules and boundaries via a mechanism called feedback. Feedback from inside and outside the system is received and processed by the person within the family who has this role. This feedback is then incorporated by the family. In the example given, the family may be very subtle in their dislike of Junior's girlfriend because they have processed how socially and politically uncomfortable explicit dislike would or could be.

The rules of the family need to be learned by you. Explicit rules will be easier (e.g., the children call all older people by their surnames), and others will be more difficult. It will be your challenge to figure out which of these rules are hindering changes within the family system and what you will do about it. What a treatment plan!

Families watch what is going on around them, specifically that which affects them. This means you: your actions, your dress, and your habits. Pay close attention to yourself. Because a family is a system, all actions serve a purpose. In isolation, Junior's behavior may be a mystery. There seems to be no trigger that you can identify while he is living residentially. A visit with Junior and his family illustrates a different context for this acting out: It occurs just as Mom and Dad begin to raise their voices in a heated discussion. One of our goals is to figure out what purpose the action serves and from this the need which is being met.

Everyone in a family has a role. Scapegoat, peacemaker, negotiator, good kid, mother, son, bad kid, gatekeeper, and speaker are some roles with which you may be familiar. Some roles are assigned automatically according to age or gender. Others are assigned according to social status or personality character-istics.

When working with families, it is important to identify to yourself who plays what role. Through the course of intervention, these roles may change. Individuals within healthy systems have roles that are fluid and dynamic. One person does not always occupy the same role. Let us say that Mom has always made arrangements for your time with the family, perhaps to the extent that if she is not home and Dad answers the phone he takes a message and suggests he will get mom to call back. This might indicate that Mom is the gatekeeper, the information gatherer, and maybe the communicator. Over time, if this is indic-ative of the problematic behaviors as identified by the family, you may begin to challenge these roles, and it would be ideal if Dad began to accept the calls and make arrangements.

Fortunately, families are open systems. This means that they are adaptive and goal-directed and therefore have the potential to find solutions and affect change. If we did not believe this, there would be no point in working with families. We have to believe in change. It is essential to doing what we do with respect and honesty.

The youngest daughter of one family came to live in our residential pro-gram. She was quickly transitioned back into the family home, and supports were provided for the family in order that they could continue to live together with less stress. One evening I visited during supper, because the father called and asked me to. He said things were going well, but they could use some sup-port.

When I arrived, the daughter, Missy, met me at the door. Her face was red, and she appeared to have been arguing: "Tell her; tell her to let me go." Appar-ently, Missy wanted to go into the city with her new boyfriend overnight to be with him when he went to a medical appointment, and Mom and Dad said no! Missy was almost 16 and they did not think that it was appropriate for her to go without a chaperone. By the time I had arrived, the fight between Missy and her mother had been going for eight hours. Missy asked permission on her way out the door to school, and when her mother refused to permit it, she decided to stay home from school to continue arguing with her mother.

There was good reason for Missy to stay and argue. The pattern several months before this would have included Missy arguing with her mother, irri-tating, threatening, and intimidating until Mom changed her mind. Before we began our work together, it only took 5 or 10 minutes for Mom to give in. After several years of Missy's harassment, Mom was exhausted and was no longer up to a fight.

On this particular day, Mom had stood her ground for eight hours! Mom used strategies like locking herself in her bedroom, wearing a walkman around the house so she could not hear Missy screaming, going for a walk with her friend, and ignoring Missy as she followed behind yelling. When Dad came home from work, he began supper so Mom would not have to be around Missy. Missy began trying to get Dad on her side, much like she did with me when I arrived. Dad deferred back to Mom and stated his support.

When I arrived, after ensuring everything was safe and getting an understanding of the situation, I began to help in the kitchen with supper. I peeled potatoes and scrubbed carrots. I chatted with Dad about past arguments with Missy. Missy joined us occasionally but spent most of her time while we were preparing supper pouting in the living room.

Missy was able to join us for supper. Her mother asked that she not argue during supper, and Missy respected that request. Conversation during supper was minimal. I struggled with my own comfort about the silences. After supper Mom explained to Missy that she was no longer going to listen to the yelling. She had made her decision, and it was to be respected. Missy looked taken aback, and ran crying to her room. Mom retired to the living room. It was peaceful; the storm had gone out to sea. Dad and I began the dishes. While we were washing the dishes, Dad commented that Missy's world would feel upside down tonight. I inquired why. He went on to explain that not only had Mom not given in, he was doing the dishes.

THE ADJUSTMENT (YOU TO THEM AND THEY TO YOU)

What meaning will families make from your behavior? This is something you need to think about. Working with families within their own home takes intentionality to another level. Not only are you working with children, you are working with and caring for the children that belong to the parents with whom you are visiting. Your behavior while in their home is the foundation for the perception they will form of you and perhaps of the program in which you are working.

The first time I went to visit the Smith family during the summer months, I had not thought about my footwear until I was at the door. While knocking, I looked down at my feet. Sandals! What now? I had already knocked, so I could not just pretend that I had not been there and reschedule for another day; I had a very important decision to make. Wear them in the house or take them off and go barefoot. The general culture in this home was to leave your shoes and coat in the entry hallway. What would I do about sandals?

Perhaps this seems like a rather odd question. Still, it represents *all* that working with families means. It means letting go of many of our own values and beliefs, recognizing that we are doing that, and accepting their value and belief system. We are shedding our sandals and wearing our bare feet in a stranger's home. How does that feel? If it feels okay to us does that mean it feels okay to the people who own this home? If they ask us to put our sandals back on, how does that feel? Has our choice been rejected, thus rejecting us? And what are the impacts if this is true? How do we regroup to continue to work effectively with this family?

When you begin to think about including parents and families with the children who are living residentially, there are many questions that come up. How do you incorporate this many people into a treatment plan? How do you program while keeping all these individuals in mind. When you have to challenge a parent, and you will (challenging or confronting is part of the helping cycle), how can you be sure you are not unnecessarily imposing your values and beliefs on them? How do you stay consistent with the values and beliefs of the program?

The silence during supper at Missy's house made me uncomfortable, but it was much needed after a day of almost constant yelling. My need for conversation was irrelevant. My opinion about the appropriateness of Missy going with her boyfriend overnight was also irrelevant. How did I maintain focus during the chaos? The same way that we maintain focus on a daily basis while working residentially: The program I work in believes that parents should parent their children. I was there as a youth care worker, not as the parent, and this family had a treatment plan. It was my responsibility to support them in being different in relationship with each other and to work towards living together more effectively with less stress.

BEING WITH–AND IN–RELATIONSHIP

It is very important to have a supportive team. First, your teammates will keep you on task. Second, written intervention or treatment plans for a family will give you a guide with which to check in. Are your interventions consistent with those outlined in the treatment plan? Having an understanding of your boundaries in relationships is important in family work.

Being with families means being available to them, especially when they are struggling. It means having a schedule that allows you to be with them when they are doing those activities that are stressful for them.

Youth and family workers are with families when times are tough. If getting up and off to school in the morning is a struggle, perhaps the youth care and family worker will be available for the family to provide support during this time. Being with a family while they are struggling is dynamic; it does not occur on schedule. It is not simply showing up when the heat is on. It is about knowing the culture of the family. It is developing relationships, knowing patterns, and sensing rhythms (Krueger, 1991).

Child and youth care workers must be engaged in a therapeutic relationship. We do not do therapy. However, every single interaction must be based on a therapeutic framework. Thus the first goal is to establish a relationship. It is also within this relationship that we are challenged and grow ourselves (Fewster, 1990; Shaw, 1997).

These relationships are developed in much the same way as we develop relationships with the children with whom we work in residential care (Shaw, 2002): Hanging out and sharing experiences. Spending time in a family home is not all about crisis. It is also not always about intervening. This hanging out skill that we hone in the residential program is useful in a family home.

At times we hang out to see what is going on and perhaps to be there with the individual members if there is a crisis. Other times we are just there: eating supper, folding laundry, doing homework, washing dishes. What is the therapeutic value of folding the laundry? Perhaps it is the rhythmicity (Maier, 1992) or taking advantage of an opportunity to not be the guest. Perhaps it is identifying to a parent that you notice they are paying attention to different parenting responsibilities or perhaps modeling a way of being together.

When do we stop being company? How do we read the subtle cues of this family so we know when it is okay to get our own coffee? Or to get coffee for someone else? For example, it may be when you are no longer greeted at the door, that occasion when there is simply a bellow, "Come in!" Or you move from the kitchen to the living room during visits, or from the living room to the kitchen.

You may orchestrate these occurrences when the timing is right. How do you know it is right? You have to listen to yourself and others. That timing you have honed within the residential program will serve you well when you move to working with youngsters and families within the community.

You must have colleagues who will challenge you to follow intervention and treatment plans. Colleagues will keep you focused on what is going on for you when you are working with families. Just as when you are working within a residential framework, you will have to work through what is evoked emotionally for you and decide how you are going to process these issues so that you can still be effective. Youth care and family work means constantly balancing your business with the business of the family and children you are working with.

YOUR OWN BUSINESS

What happens when the values and beliefs of a family differ from those identified by the residential program or from those you hold as an individual? Individual values and beliefs should have been worked through long before you move from within the residential program to the community to work with families. This is the job of your supervisor and your colleagues. They should challenge you in such a way that you can process your belief system and incorporate those that are valued by the program into your working style. Your own belief system may include values that are not appreciated by a program or family. You have to determine if you are going to let go of these or how you are going to let go of these and how you will ensure they are not inflicted on the families and children with whom you work. I once worked with a youngster who collected knives. As a program we did not value violence, and knife collecting seemed to be associated with violence. When time was spent with the family, it became clear that collecting knives had cultural significance to them. One of the parents had a first-nation heritage and identified collecting knives as part of their harvesting rituals. Our challenge then became supporting the youngster to translate his collecting of knives as a weapon and melding it with his parents' beliefs and values. As a residential program we had to come to a middle ground with our opinions and perhaps our stereotypes about weapons and the use of them.

How do you engage a family to work with a CYC program that is family focused? Well, how do you engage a child to work with a youth care program? It is activities and experiences that engage them. It is dynamic youth care and family workers. It is people who have the ability to be with them and not judge them, teach them without intruding, and care about them unconditionally. You have to take the time to establish a relationship with parents and children before you begin any "work." Entering a family home and deciding within minutes that you will challenge their parenting style is likely going to be a turn-off. Do not be surprised if you are greeted with behavior that you interpret as avoidance the next time you approach this family.

What happens when you are working with a family with whom you find it difficult to empathize? Empathy is not a universally understood word and is often misused. Empathy is the ability to understand the feelings of the youngster or family and to communicate to them that you understand what they are feeling. We do not have to agree with or accept these feelings. It is important to accept the individual, but it is not necessary to always approve of how they are feeling. When reflecting what you have heard it is important to do so without inserting your own judgments to the meaning you have made. If you are thinking that a parent is not wanting to spend time with their child, and they are explaining why, it is necessary to reflect what they have said, not what you think. The time may come later to challenge this explanation.

Working with a family with whom you struggle is a bit different than working with a youngster within the residential program who you find difficult. This difficulty may be personality, or it may be that they present a behavior that you interpret as sabotaging your interventions and work with them. When you work with a youngster like this, you often have a team of youth care workers to directly share your experiences. Working with a family in isolation from the youth-care team does not afford this luxury. It is still important to rely on your teammates. They have knowledge and experiences to share even though they are not directly involved with the family. They are also on the outside and can sometimes see the forest for the trees. Sometimes they may be able to identify for you the personal issues when you cannot specifically see it.

While people hear what they need to hear and make meaning of an interaction or experience through their own lens (Ricks, 1989), it is still important to be clear in your choice of words when reflecting back to a parent or youngster what you have understood them to say. When a parent is struggling with their children and is perhaps feeling defeated and unworthy, an empathetic response grounded in true caring has the potential to cement a connection within a therapeutic framework.

CONCLUDING COMMENTS

It is not our responsibility to determine if children are "bad" or if parents are "unfit." Leave that to the professionals who have chosen those jobs. Our responsibility is to engage in a relationship with parents and children that may facilitate change and allows them to live together more effectively with less stress. We are not social workers or psychologists. We get the great job of spending time getting to know people at a level not available to other professions. We get to be with families while they are being families. We may be there for birthdays and holidays or simpler family rituals like rent-a-movie night. We support parents while they tuck their children into bed and play with games with them, read to them, and cuddle them.

In order to be accepted by other professionals, we have to identify ourselves as professionals. We have to value our job and know the theory associated with it. We have to know our history and appreciate it. We have to be able to talk the walk and walk the talk, both with other professionals and with other youth care workers. Understanding the CYC approach and what makes it unique is part of the task, but maintaining that focus when we are alone, away from the residential unit, being with a family can be difficult.

Not everyone should do family work. A CYC worker must be well grounded in the theory of youth care, the values and beliefs of the residential program, and in touch with oneself. It is a supervisor's responsibility to identify when a youth care worker is at the stage of professional growth (Garfat, 2001; Hill, 1989; Phelan, n.d.) that will allow them to work effectively in the community without direct supervision. As a CYC worker we need to know how these stages have been defined so that we can intelligently and eloquently advocate for responsibilities with our supervisors. We need to know so that we can understand what our supervisor is talking about so that we do not accept or advocate responsibilities that we are not ready for developmentally.

Working with families requires CYC staff and program supervisors to be educated in a variety of family theories, an understanding of how family work will impact on the residential program (see, for example, Hill, this issue), and a clear grounding in youth care theory and practice. For child and youth care workers who are grounded in the residential unit, there is no better arena to hone interventions that use daily life events for therapeutic purposes (Garfat, 1995). Once grounded, they can branch out. This branching out may include working with families and, when it does, a whole new professional role is exposed.

REFERENCES

Fewster, G. (1990). *Being in child care: A journey into self.* New York: The Haworth Press, Inc.

Fewster, G., & Garfat, T. (1993). Residential child and youth care. In C. Denholm, R. Ferguson, & A. Pence (Eds.), *Professional child and youth care* (2nd ed., pp. 9-36), Vancouver, BC: University of British Columbia Press.

Garfat, T. (1995). Everyday life opportunities for impactful child and youth care. *Journal of Child and Youth Care, 10*(2), v-viii.

Garfat, T. (1998). The effective child and youth care intervention. *Journal of Child and Youth Care, 12*(1-2), 1-168.

Garfat, T (1999, September). On hanging-out and hanging-in. *CYC-Online, 8.* Retrieved January 22, 2003, from *http://www.cyc-net.org/cyc-online/cycol-0999-editorial.html*

Garfat, T. (2001, January). Developmental stages of child and youth care workers: An interactional perspective. Retrieved January 22, 2003, from *http://www.cyc-net.org/cyc-online/cycol-0101-garfat.html*

Garfat, T. (2003, March). Four parts magic: The anatomy of a child and youth care intervention. Available online from *http://www.cyc-net.org/cyc-online/cycol-0303-thom.html*

Garfat, T., & McElwee, N. (2001). The changing role of family in child and youth care practice. *Journal of Child and Youth Care Work, 15-16,* 236-248.

Hill, M., & Garfat. T. (2003). Moving to youth care family work in residential programs: A supervisor's perspective on making the transition. *Child & Youth Services,* 25(1/2), 211-223.

Hills, M. D. (1989). The child and youth care student as an emerging professional practitioner. *Journal of Child and Youth Care,* 4(1), 17-31.

Kruger, M. (1991). Coming from your center, being there, teaming up, meeting them where they're at, interacting together, counseling on the go, etc.: Central themes in professional child and youth care. *Journal of Child and Youth Care,* 5(1), 77-87.

Kwantes, C. (1992). Rethinking residential care: Working systemically within the constraints of residential treatment. *Journal of Child and Youth Care,* 7(3), 33-44.

Maier, H. W. (1992). Rhythmicity–A powerful force for experiencing unity and personal connections. *Journal of Child and Youth Care Work, 5,* 7-13.

Minuchin, S. (1974). *Families and family therapy.* Cambridge, MA: Harvard University Press.

Phelan, J. (n.d.). Stages of child and youth care worker development. Retrieved January 21, 2003, from *http://www.cyc-net.org/phelanstages.html*

Ricks, F. (1989). Self-awareness model for training and application in child and youth care. *Journal of Child and Youth Care,* 4(1), 33-42.

Shaw, K. (1997). Rethinking Christmas. *Journal of Child and Youth Care,* 11(4), 85-88.

Shaw, K. (2002 May). CYC Online. Retrieved January 25, 2003, from *http://www. cycnet.org/cyc-online/cycol-0502-kelly.html*

Whittaker, J. (1979). *Caring for troubled youth.* San Francisco: Jossey-Bass.

Interactive Youth and Family Work

Mark Krueger

SUMMARY. Youthwork and family work are similar processes of human interaction. As youthworkers, youth, and family members move through a day or shift or visit, they learn and grow together. The goal is to create as many moments of connection, discovery, and empowerment as possible. *[Article copies available for a fee from The Haworth Document Delivery Service: 1-800-HAWORTH. E-mail address: <docdelivery@haworthpress.com> Website: <http://www.HaworthPress.com> © 2003 by The Haworth Press, Inc. All rights reserved.]*

KEYWORDS. Youthwork with families, youth care work, social work with families, family-centered residential care, child and youth care, family services, family support, parent education, residential care work and families

INTRODUCTION

A basic premise for this volume is that youth workers do both youth and family work and that they have a way unique to them of doing the latter. There are several orientations to a discussion of this nature. For example, youth and family work might be thought of as distinctly different processes: A youth worker would do youth work with youth and family work with families. Or youth and family work might be seen as being intertwined. The youth worker would do some family work with youth and some youth work with families.

Another orientation, which is the one explored here, is that youth and family work are similar processes of interaction: a way of being *in* the lived experi-

Mark Krueger is affiliated with the University of Wisconsin-Milwaukee.

[Haworth co-indexing entry note]: "Interactive Youth and Family Work." Krueger, Mark. Co-published simultaneously in *Child & Youth Services* (The Haworth Press, Inc.) Vol. 25, No. 1/2, 2003, pp. 55-65; and: *A Child and Youth Care Approach to Working with Families* (ed: Thom Garfat) The Haworth Press, Inc., 2003, pp. 55-65. Single or multiple copies of this article are available for a fee from The Haworth Document Delivery Service [1-800-HAWORTH, 9:00 a.m. - 5:00 p.m. (EST). E-mail address: docdelivery@haworthpress.com].

ence *with* youth and families that promotes their development and changes or enhances their stories and patterns of interaction. The following examples will serve as a foundation for the discussion.

Bedtime

It is approaching bedtime at Nexus, a group home for troubled teens. Nicole is working. Six youth are scurrying about, teasing her and each other, and trying to give her a rough time. She sits them down and reminds them of a conversation they had earlier about the expectations for bedtime and asks them to reflect a moment on how they are behaving.

As they begin their bedtime chores, Nicole stays closer to those youth who seem to need her the most as she passes a tube of toothpaste or bar of soap or hands a towel to someone in the shower. Her voice is friendly and steady–and firm when it needs to be.

She dims the lights, lowers the music, sets pajamas on the beds in the three double rooms, and picks up after a girl who is quite capable of doing it for her self but tonight needs a little extra care.

She encourages some to speed up a little and others to slow down. Once they are in their rooms, she gauges the amount of closeness and attention each youth receives. One youth needs a moment to talk quietly, another the covers pulled up to her chin, and another just a friendly goodnight. Some want the shades down and the door closed while others want the shade up, with just a slight crack in the door to let in the light from the hallway.

Family Visit

As Nicole parks the car and walks to the house, she tries to get a feel for the surroundings. She rings the doorbell and takes a deep breath. One of the drapes is pulled aside. She catches a glimpse of someone who could be the mother. The woman opens the door and steps aside, motioning for Nicole to come in without saying anything.

"I'm John's mother–have a seat," the woman says.

"Thank you." Nicole sits on the edge of the couch.

"I was just doing the dishes."

"Can I give you a hand?" Nicole asks.

The mother pauses, seemingly surprised by the offer, then says, "If you'd like."

They work together. As they talk, the mother passes the dishes to Nicole to dry.

MOMENTS OF CONNECTION, DISCOVERY AND EMPOWERMENT

In both examples, Nicole tries, as she does in most other situations in youth and family work, to develop relationships and support the development and well-being of the youth and the mother. She listens, is genuine, lends a helping hand, and so forth. The goal, one can argue, is to create as many moments of connection, discovery, and empowerment as possible. These moments fuel development. Youth and family members, in other words, are more likely to change and grow when they feel connected to others, discover something about themselves and the world around them, and feel empowered to move forward.

In youth as well as family work, a moment of human connection occurs when Nicole, the youth, and/or the mother are in the moment together, engaged with each other and/or the task at hand. There is a sense that we are here, you and I, in our activity with one another. Nicole, for example, connects with the youth as she helps them get ready for bed, or with the mother as they do dishes. Nicole listens to a mother or youth, her attention focused on them. She is open and available to mirror back her experience of the youth and mother (Fewster, 1999).

During these moments, they are in synch, emotionally and physically, their feelings and movements more or less in harmony. The emotional and physical space is just right. "It feels good to be in this place as we interact." This is our place. We belong here. Our tone, mood, and tempo have created a safe place, a place of warmth, acceptance, and encouragement.

Usually what they are doing has meaning or a sense of purpose. It is not a chore but a task they can do together that is meaningful. Nicole works with a group of youth and parents on a clean-up project. They work together at a steady pace, sharing a sense of conviction about doing and completing the task.

Sometimes, however, they are just simply in the moment with no intended purpose. They are there, and it is simply good to be there with each other with no intended purpose other than to be together.

A moment of discovery occurs when a worker or youth or parent has an "aha" or "I got it" experience. He or she figures something out, solves a problem, or understands a feeling in a way that he or she has not.

Nicole encourages discussion. She wants the group or family to explore different sides of an issue before making a decision. The pros and cons of a home visit for a youth are discussed, and the alternatives weighed until the parents can figure out what is best for the youth and family.

Nicole helps youth and parents master the basics and then advance to more complex interventions. She presents increasingly more complex tasks and problems. For example, the simple technique of listening is important in and of itself, but it is even more effective when parents understand what it means to be in the moment and really hear what they are saying to each other.

With Nicole's assistance, a parent who feels that being consistent is crucial to disciplining youth begins to discover that most situations occur in unique contexts and that certain disciplines work in one context but not another. Nicole, for example, suggests to a father that the next time he corrects his son's behavior it might be better to do it privately rather than in front of his siblings. Or Nicole sits on a piano bench next to a boy who is learning to improvise as he plays the piano. Each new chord combination seems to open the way for new possibilities. As he tests out these possibilities he also begins to refine his technique and recognize patterns of playing that run through his choices.

A moment of empowerment occurs when a youth or parent says or feels, "I can do it. I feel good about myself. I am worthy of the task at hand." In a gymnastics activity, Nicole walks beside a boy, holding his hand as the youth tries to traverse a balance beam. At first the boy wobbles a bit using her hand for support. After a few steps his confidence grows, and the worker lets go of his hand, realizing that if he moves a little faster he is less likely to lose his balance. On a family visit at the agency Nicole has the youth demonstrate for his father, then invites the father to give it a try.

Nicole shows a mother how to get her son up in the morning with a friendly, insistent tone of voice. The mother gives it a try. With a group of youth and parents, Nicole works on several math problems, each problem using the same formula. They are fully engaged together in trying to solve the problems. Nicole provides clues along the way, and then they get it and begin to work alone on the problems.

A girl who is afraid of heights climbs a hill with her mother and Nicole. "That wasn't so bad," the girl says. A boy who is afraid to ask a girl out for a date talks with Nicole and his father to build his courage; then he calls the girl.

PRACTICES

To create these moments in youth and family work Nicole uses several practices. First, with an awareness of *developmental dynamics* (Maier, 1987) she tries to gear her interactions to the unique needs and strengths of each participant. She constantly asks herself, "Where is this youth/parent at emotionally, socially, cognitively and physically, and how can I best interact with sensitivity to their needs and strengths? Based on their prior experiences, what are they thinking? How have they learned to interact? Are they physically well?" Then she responds with sensitivity to a youth or parent's developmental capacity and/or readiness to participate. She pushes for a new insight or challenges them to participate in a new activity. The time is right to talk about their feelings or to work together on solving a problem.

As she interacts, Nicole is also aware that each person has a unique story and that no two people see a situation through the same lens. Each person has a unique perspective. Thus, she *makes meaning* by talking with the mother and youth about their experiences (Bruner, 1990; Garfat, 1998). "This is what it's like for me. What's it like for you?" she asks as searches for a mutual reality or a common place from which they can understand and be with one another and open the door for self-discovery or for finding the solution to a problem. "Now I see," the youth or mother says.

Nicole also tries to *act with purpose* (Bruner, 1990). Her actions and words say or suggest that making beds, talking, and doing dishes are the most meaningful thing they can do together at that time. She *listens*. She gives youth and family members her undivided attention. She is *present* (Fewster, 1990, 1999) in the moment. Her eyes are alert and attentive. There is a sense that I am here, fully in this moment, for you and myself, and with enthusiasm for the task at hand.

She has *empathy*. She is curious and sincere in her desire to know the other person. They see in her a sense of self-awareness that has opened her to being there for them.

Their *rhythmic interactions* permeate their moments together and "forge human connections" (Maier, 1992, p. 7). A youth and Nicole run together, sharing a common pace. Or Nicole works side-by-side with the youth and the mother as they get ready for bed or do dishes with sensitivity to the tempo of the conversation, the movement of their bodies and hands, and the nods of their heads. The pace and tone of their interactions are in harmony. They are not moving too fast or too slow. She changes the rhythm or tempo to increase the pace of conversation or action or to provide the necessary impetus a youth or the mother needs to gain a new insight or skill.

As she moves through the day, Nicole gets a feel for the group and senses where she is in *proximity* (Redl & Wineman, 1952, p. 164) to others. She adjusts her position and moves closer or farther away from a youth. At one moment she is in the center of the group, leading, and in another moment she is at the edge, following. An upbeat tempo is required or things need to be slowed down. She adjusts her movement and position accordingly.

She adjusts the atmosphere to support their interactions: a large space for a game or a small space for a talk. With sensitivity to how youth and the mother feel or act, she guides them to a public or private place, or to a personal or unfamiliar place. She raises or dims the lights, turns the music up or down, acts upbeat or serious.

There are, of course, many more similar practices in youth and family work. These are just a few. The point is that youth and family work are similar process of interactions in which workers try to be *in* their interactions *with* youth and family members as they try to create moments of connection, discovery, and empowerment.

THE DYNAMICS OF GROUPS AND FAMILIES

The dynamics of groups and families are similar in many ways. Families, like groups, are large and small and comprised of various combinations of individuals, each of whom plays a unique role in the group or family. Members of groups and families develop unique patterns of interaction. In some families and groups, the members might openly express their feelings; whereas in other groups and families the members are more reserved.

Some group and family patterns of interaction are harmful. Abusive families or groups develop patterns of denial, hurt, and rejection. Or in some families, the parents without knowing it–or for what they think are good reasons–criticize or punish their children in ways that leave emotional scars.

Groups or families have different influences on each participant depending on a number of circumstances. In some situations youth try to be like their parents and peers, and in other situations they try to be different. The meaning of group and family influences is also constantly changing. Each new experience in youthwork and life adds a new layer of meaning to the youth's sense of self and the influences family and peers have on the development of that sense of self. In any given moment or interaction, the role of the family or peers in influencing a youth's behavior and feelings might be a major or minor factor with any number of other factors contributing to a situation.

Nicole's role with groups and families is similar to the process described a moment ago. Her goal is to create as many moments of connection, discovery, and empowerment as possible. She is sensitive to presence, rhythm, meaning, and atmosphere as it applies to each individual. She gets a sense of where the family as a whole is in the midst of a discussion or a task as well as where each individual is in the process. She feels where she is in relationship to the family members and their need for closeness or distance and shifts her position or directs her comments, trying to engage each person.

For example, Nicole sits down to eat with the youth in the group home, aware that mealtimes have a different meaning for each youth. For one youth the meal evokes memories of a time when dad came home drunk and argued with mom. In another youth's home, often there was not enough to eat. Another youth ate alone in front of the TV.

She makes eye contact with a youth as he or she passes the fried beans, extending her hand as if to connect with a youth for a moment. "Try it, I think you will like it," she says. As they eat she is present with sensitivity to the tone and tempo of the meal.

Similarly, she sits with a family having dinner while listening and observing. She is aware that their individual experiences of what is about to occur are different than her experience. She also knows the family has a history of eating together and that they have developed unique patterns of interaction at meals and elsewhere. As they talk, she searches for opportunities to connect. She also looks for opportunities to help family members discover solutions to their own problems and feel empowered. At one point she suggests to the father that perhaps there is another way to get a youth off to school in the morning, and the father says, "Yes, perhaps if I wake him up earlier it will be less of a struggle." Or, she gives the mother a phone number to enroll her daughter in a computer class.

LEARNING TO DANCE

To engage successfully in this process, Nicole learns her craft and brings herself to the moment. She educates herself and tries to understand her own stories and practices. She learns to listen and to be present. She also learns to plan and conduct interactions and activities according to developmental (social, emotional, cognitive, physical, and spiritual) needs and strengths and with sensitivity to the multiple meanings that interactions, environments, and activities have for youth and family members.

Needless to say, this is a challenging approach to youth and family work. One has to have self-awareness and sensitivity to the developmental strengths and needs of each youth and family member, curiosity about each person's unique story, and an awareness of how any number of factors influence the contexts within which interactions occur. It requires experience, knowledge, and technical skill. It also requires the capacity to think on your feet and to improvise to the tempos of daily living.

I find it helpful to think of youth workers as modern dancers, that is, those who perform as part of a dance troupe on stage or professional dancers who choreograph a dance and then improvise on stage to the music (Krueger, 1998,

2002). Like modern dancers, workers try to use their intuition and instincts as well as their knowledge in their interactions. They get a feel for what is occurring as much as they have an objective awareness.

Their movements, the tone and tempo of their actions, and their positions are as important as their thoughts about what they are doing. For example, Nicole enters a youth's home or bedroom at the group home. Using her knowledge and prior experience, she simultaneously senses where she should be in relationship to the family members or the youth, how close or far, and the impact of the atmosphere, the mood, tone, tempo and physical nature of the surroundings. She steps forward or back, sits down or stands, and comments or does not comment on what she sees based on how she reads and feels about the situation.

A modern dance instructor I invited to teach part of my youthwork class told me that in modern dance there are two fundamental movements: lining up and passing through. Dancers line up with one another and or pass through or between each other. Similarly, Nicole tries to get a feel for where she is in relationship to family members. She lines up and passes through these spaces while getting a feel for when to be close or far and mirroring back her experience of them.

Thus the competent youth and family worker knows and senses how to move and where to be in relationship to youth and family members as he or she tries to create moments of connection, discovery, empowerment. He or she gets a feel for the circumstance and the people in it and tries to orchestrate a story. There is a time to use self to change the tempo, a time to pull back, a time to be close, moments when an increase in pace and the volume of the music will best serve a situation, and moments when quiet and stillness will work better. At the same time they try to be in the moment, fully involved in their activity. They are not consumed by the past or future, fully in the experience of doing and being with a youth or family member.

Their goal throughout the dance is to contribute moments that will enrich the youths' and families' stories. This is not always an easy process. There is as much if not more struggle than success. Youth and family members with habits of interacting are often slow to give these up, because they have in some way served them well as means of avoidance and/or defense against pain. Further, change is often not recognizable until later when the participants in an interaction have a moment to reflect on what has occurred. What they do together during the dance lingers and slowly takes hold when they interact in new situations. A youth or parent says, "Ah, now I see. That makes sense." Sometimes it is just the experience of being together that counts. It occurs and is forgotten, but at least it has occurred, and the participants have experienced it.

In closing it might be helpful to take another look now at the examples presented at the beginning and explore how Nicole dances. For the purpose of discussion, an additional family member has been added to the second example.

Bedtime

It is approaching bedtime at Nexus, a group home for troubled teens. Nicole is working. Six youth are scurrying about, teasing her and each other, and trying to give her a rough time. She sits them down and reminds them of a conversation they had earlier about the expectations for bedtime and asks them to reflect a moment on how they are behaving.

As they begin their bedtime chores, Nicole stays closer to those youth who seem to need her the most as she passes a tube of toothpaste or bar of soap or hands a towel to someone in the shower. Her voice is friendly and steady and firm when it needs to be.

She dims the lights, lowers the music, sets pajamas on the beds in the three double rooms, and picks up after a girl who is quite capable of doing it for herself but tonight needs a little extra care.

She encourages some to speed up a little and others to slow down. Once they are in their rooms, she gauges the amount of closeness and attention each youth receives. One youth needs a moment to talk quietly, another the covers pulled up to her chin, and another just a friendly goodnight. Some want the shades down and the door closed while others want the shade up, with just a slight crack in the door to let the light from the hallway shine through.

Family Visit

Nicole makes a home visit to meet the family of a new boy at the group home. As she parks the car and walks to the house, she tries to get her own feel for the surroundings. She rings the doorbell and takes a deep breath. One of the drapes is pulled aside. She catches a glimpse of someone who could be the mother. In a moment the woman opens the door and steps aside, motioning for Nicole to come in without saying anything.

"I'm John's mother–have a seat," the woman says.

"Thank you." Nicole sits on the edge of the couch.

"I was just doing the dishes."

"Can I give you a hand?" Nicole asks.

The mother pauses, seemingly surprised by the offer, then says, "If you'd like."

Soon they are working together, the mother passing the dishes to Nicole to dry, a rhythm developing between them as Nicole gauges the tempo and content of the conversation, trying to sense as well as know when to interject a personal question about the family and the mother's son, their actions and togetherness in the moment perhaps meaning more than the words.

The boy's sister, Maria, comes in from school, looks at Nicole inquisitively: "Who are you?"

"Nicole. I work with your brother."

"Hmm." She puts her books on the table and sits down. "How is he doing?"

"Well, he's a little lonely and angry right now."

"He should be. I don't know why they put him there anyway."

"Maria, we've been through this," the mother says.

Nicole pauses–then says, "That's okay; I'd like to hear how Maria feels," and hands Maria an extra towel.

Maria looks at Nicole, gets up, stands beside her, grabs a dish.

"I'm angry!" Maria says.

"I understand. I imagine you miss him?"

"I don't miss him. I just don't think they should have taken him away." She puts the dish on the table. Nicole hands her another one.

CONCLUSION

There are several ways to look at youth and family work. One way is to view youth and family work as a process of interaction that occurs in situations such as these when workers are in the moment with understanding and self-awareness, moving and acting in a way that will contribute to a sense of connection, discovery, and empowerment. During the process, family informs youth work and youth work informs family work. The workers knowledge and acceptance of the role of family in the lives of youth aids their ability to interact with youth, and the skills they develop as youth workers aids their ability to work with families.

This is a complex process, full of struggle and failure. When they are "on," youth workers are dancing. They sense as well as know what to do as they bring themselves to the moment, act with purpose, and try to be in synch with the youths' and family members' developmental rhythms for trusting in an atmosphere that supports growth, change, and/or just being together.

REFERENCES

Baizerman, M. (1990-present). Musing with Mike (an occasional column). *Child and Youth Care Forum.*

Bruner, J. (1990). *Acts of meaning.* Cambridge, MA: Harvard University Press.

Dejardins, S., & Freeman, A. (1991). Out of synch. *Journal of Child and Youth Care, 6,* 139-144.

Fahlberg, V. (1990). *Residential treatment: A tapestry of many therapies.* Indianapolis: Perspectives Press.

Fewster, G. (1999). Turning myself inside out: My theory of me. *Journal of Child and Youth Care, 13*, 35-54.

Fewster, G. (1990). *Being in child care: A journey into self.* New York: The Haworth Press, Inc.

Fulcher, L. (1999). The soul, rhythm, and blues of residential child care practice. *Journal of Child and Youth Care, 4*, 13-28.

Garfat, T. (1998). The effective child and youth care intervention. *Journal of Child and Youth Care, 12*, 1-178.

Guttman, E. (1991). Immediacy in residential child and youth care: The fusion of experience, self-consciousness, and action. In J. Beker & Z. Isikovits (Eds.), *Knowledge utilization in residential child and youth care practice.* Washington, DC: Child Welfare League of America.

Krueger, M. (in press). *In the rhythms of youth: Themes and stories in youth work practice.* New York: The Haworth Press, Inc.

Krueger, M. (1998). *Interactive youth work practice.* Washington, DC: Child Welfare League of America.

Krueger, M. (1995). *Nexus: A book about youth work.* Washington, DC: Child Welfare League of America.

Maier, H. (1995). Genuine child and youth care practice across the North American continent. *Journal of Child and Youth Care, 10*, 11-22.

Maier, H. (1992). Rhythmicity–A powerful force for experiencing unity and personal connections. *Journal of Child and Youth Care Work, 8*, 7-13.

Maier, H. (1987). *Development group care of children and youth: Concepts and practice.* New York: The Haworth Press, Inc.

Phelan, J. (2001). Experiential counseling and the CYC practitioner. *Journal of Child and Youth Care Work, 15-16*, 257-264.

Redl, F., & Wineman, D. (1952). *Controls from within: Techniques for the treatment of the aggressive child.* New York: Free Press.

Rose Sladde, L. (1996). Journal entries. *Journal of Child and Youth Care, 10*(4), 79-83.

Child and Youth Care Family Support Work

Jack Phelan

SUMMARY. This article describes the theoretical process and practical skills involved in a child and youth care approach to family work. The behaviors and boundary dynamics for this worker are significantly different than those envisioned in family therapy approaches, including gaining credibility by actually living with difficult youth, trusting families to know what they need, supporting families by doing useful things in the life space, having a systemic view of families, maintaining clear boundaries in an intimate environment, the use of analogue communication versus dialogue, and having an "observing ego." *[Article copies available for a fee from The Haworth Document Delivery Service: 1-800-HAWORTH. E-mail address: <docdelivery@haworthpress.com> Website: <http://www.HaworthPress.com> © 2003 by The Haworth Press, Inc. All rights reserved.]*

KEYWORDS. Youthwork with families, youth care work, social work with families, family-centered residential care, child and youth care, family services, family support, parent education, residential care work and families

What is it about a child and youth care (CYC) approach to working with families that is so unique? We should start with a basic description that informs the rest of our discussion. CYC family support work is a powerful, distinct, and

Jack Phelan is affiliated with Grant MacEwan College.

[Haworth co-indexing entry note]: "Child and Youth Care Family Support Work." Phelan, Jack. Co-published simultaneously in *Child & Youth Services* (The Haworth Press, Inc.) Vol. 25, No. 1/2, 2003, pp. 67-77; and: *A Child and Youth Care Approach to Working with Families* (ed: Thom Garfat) The Haworth Press, Inc., 2003, pp. 67-77. Single or multiple copies of this article are available for a fee from The Haworth Document Delivery Service [1-800-HAWORTH, 9:00 a.m. - 5:00 p.m. (EST). E-mail address: docdelivery@haworthpress.com].

different method of helping families to function more effectively and to acquire the competency and hopefulness that will enable them to be more successful in the future. CYC work with family as the focus will be more clearly understood as we articulate CYC work with youth.

LEARNING IN RESIDENTIAL CARE

Residential programs provide the basic training ground for many CYC professionals. In those settings, the CYC professional engages the youth by living alongside him or her, building a safe and predictable environment by "containing" injurious or irresponsible behavior that the youth may display (Winnicott, 1984). The worker engages in nurturing and caring interactions with youth who have difficulty with attachment to create safe, trustworthy relationship connections and allowing the youth to learn and grow.

CYC professionals typically reach a crossroad early in their career (usually between year 1 and 2), where they must choose between blaming parents and families and trying to rescue the youth from this influence, or seeing parents and families as partners who may also need our support to be more capable of handling their life challenges (Phelan, 2003). Good family support workers have chosen the latter path.

The experience of living day-to-day with the behaviors and beliefs of this unique population is a fertile training ground for future success with family work. The most straightforward issue is that the worker develops a tremendous respect for parents through experiencing the difficulty of living with these youth who have very challenging behavior. The more skilled worker understands how to use developmental lenses and other theories to support the youth's strengths and appreciates the complex reasons for the existing behavior.

Parents know intuitively whether the family support worker can "walk the talk" because of having actually dealt with youth similar to their own. Without at least some personal credibility, the family will have little reason to trust the worker.

A major lesson for the worker is realizing that many people get stuck in destructive patterns of living and want to live more happy lives but do not know how to change.

Associated with this lesson is learning that relationship building plays a key role in any attempt to enter a person's life-space, and change will only occur after a relationship exists. The resistance of youth and families to relationship-building attempts by well-meaning workers also begins to be appreciated and understood as a protective strategy rather than simply as a "negative behavior."

Another lesson is that most youth are protective of their family and especially of the parents. Even when youth experience tremendous relief as the difficulties in the family begin to be addressed, they defend their parents' dignity and status. Youth have idealistic views of the parents who they perhaps wished they had, and we can see the strength and beauty here rather than the need to create a more "realistic" picture.

Another, more complicated understanding emerges as CYC workers become more skilled: The worker sees the value in creating small steps toward change that are developmentally helpful, even though they may not look useful to the untrained eye. For example, workers learn to support behaviors that are not the ultimate goal but are necessary transition stages. So, for example, a youth may be encouraged to be selfish or loud and demanding in order to assist them to acquire a sense of personal power and autonomy. Youth may be supported to make mistakes and do things that are outside the usual rules in order to develop a sense of trust and self-control. These strategies can look foolish or wrong when viewed only on a short-term basis, and unskilled workers may be unable to understand these ideas. The skillful CYC worker uses a theoretical map to guide interventions and this ability to have a theoretical lens to look at behavior is crucial to good family support work.

Change occurs slowly and in many ways that are not simple and linear, and skillful workers appreciate this fact. We really do have to resist the urge to tell people what to do based on our view of the world, to allow youth and families the opportunity to create the changes.

CYC FAMILY SUPPORT WORK

The CYC approach includes the use of the family's life space and actual shared lived moments to create helpful interventions. The power of using lived experience and strategic, immediate, purposeful reflection on that experience enables CYC family support workers to facilitate shifts that simply do not occur with more passive and indirect methods. The boundaries for the workers are more intimate and less protected by professional distancing strategies such as would be typical in an office-based interview. Boundary definition is a key piece of our work, yet we must see our relationship with the family as equal, not superior. The context must honor the parent as the expert on their family, and the worker is not only not above the family in knowing what needs to be done but is even in a "one down" position. One father who had been resistant to many attempts at family therapy described finally being willing to work with a CYC worker who "didn't come into his home with a plan already formulated about what he needed to do" (Sullivan, 1995).

The work is less reliant on dialogue and therapeutic reflection and more on experiential, lived moments, often co-experienced by the family and the worker. The CYC approach has been characterized as the process of arranging experiences that challenge the family to revisit old self-defeating patterns and beliefs through the cognitive dissonance that arises as a felt experience of success; competence gets highlighted through purposeful reflection in the moment (Phelan, 1999). Workers support youth and families to feel the experience of being competent by actually doing things that are useful and capturing the moment before it evaporates.

The relationship developed between the family and worker is founded on a sense of safety that grows out of mutuality and a "non-expert" stance by the worker rather than the power relationship that occurs when a person goes to an expert to be healed. The process of CYC family support work is described by Romanko-Woods (1999) quite elegantly as a three-stage model:

- Create a safe relationship;
- Do the change work; and
- Separate and close (Romanko-Woods, 1999).

I will elaborate on these details as we proceed.

Systemic Approach

The first and most basic knowledge needed for a student or new worker is to acquire a systemic point of view. The theory of family systems is well described in many books and articles that are readily available. A competent family support worker uses tools like genograms (McGoldrick, 1985) and eco-maps (Holman, 1983) to assist family members to understand the systemic influences in their lives. Understanding the complexity of the family as a system that protects its own integrity is a vital building block.

As a supplement to this, it is useful to use practical stories as a way to embed the concepts for new practitioners.

During the day I worked with a group of 12 children, and two of these were brothers, Benny and Kenny. Benny was older by a year at 9, but Kenny often seemed older, since he was more articulate and outgoing.

Part of the program was recreation, lots of trips by subway to all parts of New York City, but the mornings were spent on reading and English skills. We used games and activities: Hangman, 20 questions, and a series of high interest books of increasing difficulty in a reading program set.

Kenny was a good reader, but Benny couldn't read at all. Both boys enjoyed being with me and we often spent extra time on reading. Benny tried very hard and even memorized a few of the easier books to impress me, but he was not able to read.

After several weeks, and because I had met their mother who was a classroom aide in the school system, I asked the boys to see if their parents would allow me to visit them at home to talk. I didn't have an elaborate plan, I was just looking for support.

When I visited them in their apartment in "the projects," I was struck with how much Benny looked like his father, while Kenny resembled his mom. The dad was a bit shy and reluctant to talk, but his wife got him to join us. He was a cab driver, who had worked hard even as a young boy in Puerto Rico and had left school very early to make a living. He stated that he had never learned to read and was obviously proud of his wife, who had completed high school. He was also proud of himself and what he had accomplished through his own hard work.

I asked him if he thought it was important for Benny to be able to read. He said that he didn't know if it was essential, since he had succeeded without this skill. His wife jumped in and said that she really wanted Benny to read, and her husband said, "OK with me, if that's what you want."

Somehow I realized that this wasn't enough, so I asked the father to decide for himself if he wanted Benny to read. He said he wasn't sure, and I asked him to take a few minutes to decide. He spent a few minutes thinking and then said, "This isn't Puerto Rico. He will need to read in New York." I asked the parents to call the boys in to join us, and the father said to Benny that he wanted him to learn how to read. We talked for a few more minutes and then I left. Benny was reading within a week (Phelan, 2001).

When working with a particular youth on a specific behavior, we can often get lost inside the immediate dynamics and ignore the much more powerful and pervasive influences that are really within our sphere of ability to utilize to create change. I am often saddened by the individually focussed efforts of some workers that totally ignore both the family and the other systems that surround all of us.

Micro, Meso, and Macro Systems

Another useful framework is Uri Bronfenbrenner's (1979) work (interpreted by others such as Garbarino, 1982) on ecosystems: family, peers, school, work, religion, and culture in our microsystem; neighborhood, career opportunities, local political environment, and so forth in our mesosystem; and economic conditions, national issues, and environmental concerns in our macrosystems. Each of us lives inside a system of close and distant relationships that influence who we are and how we behave. The worker can use Bronfenbrenner's work to support the person and family and maximize the beneficial relationships available to them and to increase the family member's effectiveness, happiness, and hope by coaching them to understand the mutual influence process that occurs. Many families who experience difficulty do not negotiate effectively within their own micro- and mesosystems, because the members have a limited, egocentric view of their connections with others. Workers can also appreciate the paradox of being inside the life space of a family at the same time they are outside of it in the role of coach. In summary, ecological theory gives the worker another, better lens to view the operation of the family in their world.

Most importantly, systemic thinking assists the worker to resist the urge to blame the parents for past and current issues, especially because many people will be encouraging the worker to do this. As we help family members to see multigenerational dynamics and their influence on the present, everyone can have the opportunity to minimize blame and start to work together. CYC work is typically focussed on individual youth, and systemic thinking challenges this limited view.

Systemic thinking as a way to view families is shared, hopefully, by all professionals who work with families, and it creates connections and opportunities for essential dialogue across disciplines.

Life-Space

The primary difference between family therapy and the basic foundation of CYC family support work is that it is life-space work (Redl & Wineman, 1952). It happens during the daily, real events of living in the moment. The worker performs his job in the much more dynamic and less structured environment created by the family in their home rather than in an office or agency space. The real work is less talking with and more doing with. The family often requires very real help in the form of physical needs and practical assistance and less cognitive reflection or verbal strategy advising. The helping occurs through lived-experience work, not reflection on prior or future behavior. Generally, families resist reflecting on past, painful issues and CYC workers see this as not particularly useful in any case, since distortion, self-protection, and learned helplessness are often the end product.

A story may illustrate this more effectively. This example was given at a workshop delivered by the Batshaw Youth Services (Montreal) CYC Family Support Program staff at the Inter-Association Child Care Conference (Maciocia, 2001).

Early one morning, a family support worker gets a call from a mother of a family on his caseload who is distressed at her teenage son's refusal to go to school, an ongoing problem. The worker visits immediately and is confronted by the son who states that there are no clean clothes to wear and he isn't going to school in dirty clothes. The parents describe that their washing machine is broken and there is no money to fix it. The worker spends some time listening and then takes a look at the washing machine. He sees what needs to be done to fix it and returns that afternoon with tools and the necessary part. As he lies on the floor on his back fixing the machine, the boy and both parents hover around watching. He spends the time fixing the washer as well as creating a discussion between the family members about the things that need to happen differently in the home. Two hours of fruitful discussion later, all is done.

This type of intervention would not be envisioned by most other professionals, yet it does describe an effective CYC approach.

Typical counseling strategies are a form of dialogue work, while we are using "analogue work": a use of experience to create sensory data in the moment that can be channeled into energy to change. (I also like the word analogue as it is used here in the technical sense of a system in which the volume or quantity of something parallels its proportionate measurement, e.g., volume of sound and voltage.) Reflection and observation are then purposefully inserted into the life-space event as a framework to challenge people to shift patterns and beliefs (Phelan, 2001). The ability to exist alongside our families and to co-experience the life situations as they occur enable CYC family support workers to understand the often complex rationales that keep families stuck and helpless.

One of my students described her work with a family that had seemingly resisted all attempts to change.

The family consisted of a mother and three small children, and the referral described a house that was dirty and chaotic. The goal for this worker, which had stymied other workers, was to get the mother to keep her home more clean and organized so that the children would have a safe environment. The worker spent several visits creating a safe relationship with the mother and trying to live alongside her as she lived her life. The obvious task of cleaning the house could have been done in a few hours, and the mother would often do this with other workers present and assisting her but could not do it on her own. This worker resisted suggesting this or commenting on the chaos, waiting for the mother to lead the way. As they were discussing things on the third or fourth visit, the mother finally stated that she really wanted to be able to "clean up this mess." The worker asked her when her life hadn't been such a mess and the mother smiled and said that once as a young teen she had won a sports trophy.

They found the trophy at the back of a closet and the mother looked at it proudly. The worker suggested to the mom that this was a real part of herself that she often forgot about and that perhaps she would want to put it somewhere in sight to remind her of her capabilities. Next visit the mother showed the worker that she had put the trophy on a small table in the hallway and the worker noticed that this table was perhaps the only clean space in the home. As they continued to meet, the mother described that when she was feeling overwhelmed, she would look at the trophy and feel better. Over the next months, the house became significantly cleaner and organized and the mother said that she no longer needed help (Lee, 1998).

Boundaries

Working in the life-space often produces anxiety, since personal safety can be a major concern. This lack of safety is also felt by the family members, and boundary setting can be an important issue for all. It is important for the worker to feel and be safe before trying to assist the family. Family support work might even be described as working without a safety net under you. The temptation is to shield yourself by assuming an expert stance and create distance between you and them.

The boundaries are much more intimate than in other helping roles and the worker is exposed in a way that people behind a one-way mirror never experience. There is no room in this work for a passive observer role, and families will challenge workers to be present by creating chaos and danger in the moment. Barking dogs, unwanted guests, angry spouses and youth, and loud television sets are all part of the process. The worker needs to model positive ways to deal with the chaos and lack of connection that is often present as family members struggle with the fear of abandonment if they change too much. The worker also starts to share the experience of "standing on the edge of the pit of emptiness" (Kapla, 1989) and can increase their own empathy for the family.

Another major boundary issue is the worker who is too intrusive and too controlling. There is a tendency to want to give advice, a practice that does not work; to focus on the problems and difficulties, which does not work; to assume that the parents do not know how to run their family, which is not true, and; to think that the family sees your interventions as helpful, which is wishful thinking. The most successful CYC family support workers are described by families two years later as "nice people who did very little, we did it all" (Sullivan, 1995).

Role of the Helper

CYC family support workers describe "one-down" or the non-expert role as most useful in supporting families to make changes. In this *living alongside* role where you are co-experiencing events, how does one manage to be deliberately and strategically helpful and still be genuinely present? Where does expertise get in the way, and when does being too friendly become a deficit? What exactly is appropriate professional demeanor in this situation?

As I enter your life-space and join you, in some ways it becomes my life space also. If I fully accept my presence in this moment, will I lose my ability to become deliberately supportive for you? Can I be present in your life-space without making it my life-space too? It is not possible to be totally neutral and unaffected (nor is it desirable), but it would be a mistake to lose focus on supporting the family as the main task. Yet if I hope to support you to live your life better, with less pain and more hope, then the place to support you is in your actual life-space. This "living with" becomes a mutual influence process, and it is important for the worker to remain both safe and helpful without being absorbed into the family's system. Supervision and peer support are essential in this work and the CYC worker needs to have a clear theory and strategy map to stay out of trouble.

CYC family support work training includes helping the worker to develop an "observing ego" that facilitates maintaining an objective view of the interpersonal dynamics that are occurring. The ability to be a reflective practitioner (Schon, 1983) is an essential skill. The worker must accept and understand his own response and be able to do the same with the family's response. It is difficult to keep issues separate at times.

To use the ecosystem, the worker can position him- or herself to be a coach to the family, supporting them to maximize the beneficial relationships available to them while not becoming another part of the micro- or mesosystem of the family. The role of helper is most strategically positioned in a way that the worker can see the family's whole ecosystem from outside and then step into it at strategic points in the life-space to be supportive. Thinking systemically enables the worker to utilize the interaction between people for maximum benefit.

CYC family support workers describe the need to nurture parents in the early stages of relationship building. Many parents have not had the experience of being nurtured as children and can behave very childishly at first. The worker can accept this need and gradually bring the parent through developmental stages to the point of being a nurturer to their family. The ultimate goal is to equalize the relationship between parent and worker and support the parent to take over. CYC work is founded on creating a caring process, and much of the preparation for the work focuses on nurturing skills, but it would be important to distinguish between the adult-child nurturing role and the adult-adult relationship that needs to eventually exist.

CONCLUSION

There are some essential building blocks in the process of becoming a competent CYC family support worker. The skilled practitioner has integrated a systemic point of view into all their assessments and observations, with all the tools available to most family work professionals. In addition, the use of the life-space and the process of co-experiencing the lived moment as fellow travelers without losing one's focus as a helper is a core skill. The ability to balance intimate boundary issues and to maintain an objective, reflective analysis of dynamics that occur as one "works without a net" requires experience and maturity.

The empathy and relational connection developed as one works with challenging families creates the ability to understand the logic of crisis dynamics that keep these family members connected through the centrifugal force of whirling around together. Skilled workers can live alongside this energy without being caught up in it and support the family to connect more safely.

One group of CYC family support workers describe how they know if other programs that they occasionally visit are using a CYC model. If the hairdos, manicures, and clothing of the other staff are too formal, they probably are not using this model.

So a list of skills would include:

- the use of the life-space of the family and a process of living alongside,
- the skill of arranging strategic experiences and using existing experiences to develop new views of competence and hope,
- use of primarily an analogue process of creating change rather than dialogue,
- maintaining a non-expert position,
- supporting families through behavior and physical resources,
- creating safe, yet intimate, boundaries,
- constant self-awareness and self-monitoring,
- having a theoretical map to determine strategies and direction, and
- using peers and supervisors for support and direction.

Again, the ultimate goal, as confirmed in at least one research study of successful CYC family support work (Sullivan, 1995), is to have the family believe that they did it themselves (Sullivan, 1995).

REFERENCES

Bronfenbrenner, U. (1979). *The ecology of human development*, Cambridge, MA: Harvard University Press.
Garbarino, J. (1982). *Children and families in the social environment*. New York: Norton.

Holman, A. (1983). *Family assessment: Tools for understanding and intervention*. New York: Sage.

Kagan, R. (1995). *Turmoil to turning points*. New York: Norton.

Kagan, R., & Schlosberg, S. (1989). *Families in perpetual crisis*. New York: Norton.

Lee, D. (1998). Field placement journal entry. Grant MacEwan College, Edmonton, Alberta.

Maciocia, A. (2001). *Workshop presentation on CYC family support work*. Inter-Association Child Care Conference, Valley Forge, PA.

McGoldrick, M. (1985). *Genograms in family assessment*. New York: Norton.

Phelan, J. (2003). The relationship boundaries that control programming. *Relational Child and Youth Care Practice, 16*(1), 51-56.

Phelan, J. (2001, September). My introduction to family systems theory. *CYC-On-Line, 32*.

Phelan, J. (2001). Experiential counseling and the CYC practitioner. *Journal of Child and Youth Care Work, 15-16*, 256-263.

Phelan, J. (1999). Experiments with experience. *Journal of Child and Youth Care Work, 14*, 25-28.

Redl, F., & Wineman, D. (1952). Controls from within for the treatment of the aggressive child. New York: The Free Press.

Romanko-Woods, M. (1999). *Classroom lecture notes*. Grant MacEwan College, Edmonton, Alberta.

Schon, D. (1983). *The reflective practitioner: How professionals think in action*. New York: Basic Books.

Sullivan, J. (1995). Unpublished doctoral dissertation. University of Virginia, USA.

Winnicott, D. W. (1984). *The child, the family, and the outside world*. London: Penguin.

My Place or Yours?
Inviting the Family into Child
and Youth Care Practice

Gerry Fewster

SUMMARY. Child and youth care professionals often focus on individual youth and relegate the family to a peripheral place in the work. Yet the family remains the foundation for most growth and development of youth. Working from the point of view of the subjective experience of the child allows the worker to include the family as a vehicle for change and as a fundamental aspect of child and youth care practice.

KEYWORDS. Youthwork with families, youth care work, social work with families, family-centered residential care, child and youth care, family services, family support, parent education, residential care work and families

A PERSONAL PROLOGUE

Once upon a time I worked as a family therapist at a large residential treatment center for "emotionally disturbed" children. Actually, I talked my way

Gerry Fewster is affiliated with Malaspina University College.

This article was originally published in the *Journal of Child and Youth Care*, Vol. 15(4), 137-150. It is reprinted here with the permission of the author and publisher.

[Haworth co-indexing entry note]: "My Place or Yours? Inviting the Family into Child and Youth Care Practice." Fewster, Gerry. Co-published simultaneously in *Child & Youth Services* (The Haworth Press, Inc.) Vol. 25, No. 1/2, 2003, pp. 79-94; and: *A Child and Youth Care Approach to Working with Families* (ed: Thom Garfat) The Haworth Press, Inc., 2003, pp. 79-94.

into the job when one of the program directors let it slip that they were becoming concerned about the number of children who seemed to "regress" after returning home to their families. Based on no evidence whatsoever I told him that the family will always be a far more powerful learning context than any treatment program, so if their work with the child was to have long-term benefits, they would need to include the family in their treatment designs. Strange as it may seem now, this was a fairly radical idea back in 1968. The next day, I had a call from the Executive Director and began work the following week. If anyone had asked me what a family therapist actually did, I would have been hard pressed to come up with an answer.

Later that year I went off to train with the inimitable Virginia Satir, and a new light shone from the heavens. The first time I watched this amazing woman work with a family, I could hardly contain myself. With prodigious presence, sensitivity, and skill, she gently invited each person to come forward, to bring their thoughts and feelings into the moment, intervening only to seek clarification or confront anyone who used the occasion to speak for–or condemn–another. And, with each authentic expression, the inner world of the family came to life, bringing tears, laughter, and so many "ahas" that I quickly lost count. What I noticed most was how the energy shifted from being stifled and shallow to open and full as the participants became increasingly animated, engaged, and alive. While my thoughts were wordless, I intuitively knew that this was what *real* change was all about; not the superficial shifts in attitude or behavior designed to satisfy external expectations or demands, but the change that comes from the undesigned spontaneous expressions of the Self–transformation and growth, *from the inside-out*. I wanted to know this woman's secrets–to learn her techniques and replicate her forms. But later, as I watched others attempt to do just this, I realized that the secret was more about Virginia herself even as, for a few months, I actually tried to be like her by mouthing her words, imitating her gestures, assimilating her attitudes, and generally trying to assume her persona. Only gradually did it dawn on me that the real secret was for me to become more like Gerry Fewster.

Now, few professionals would bother to debate my cavalier assertion that, wherever possible, a child's residential program should involve the family. It simply made sense that, since a child's attitudes and behaviors are learned in the family, any gains derived from a residential experience would quickly evaporate if the youngster is returned to an unchanged home environment. It seemed to me that there were three possible options to consider:

a. Keep the child at home and work with the family as a whole;
b. Remove the child for a brief period of respite or "treatment" and engage the family in preparing for the youngster's return; and

   c. Remove the child permanently and arrange an alternative long-term placement.

In those days there was no profession of child and youth care, but the front-line residential staff were called "child care workers."

Much as I enjoyed working with families, I found myself constantly gravitating back to the kids who had been identified as "the presenting problem." At the same time I became increasingly disenchanted with what was taking place on the family therapy bandwagon. In search of a distinct professional identity, it seemed that the new advocates of family intervention were zealously embracing a perspective that dismissed individual lives in order to focus on the family as a "system." With the tacit belief that human feelings, attitudes and behaviors are essentially responses to environmental conditions, everyone seemed to be searching for replicable interventions that could bring about desired outcomes, with the practitioner pressing the buttons–a distinctly *outside-in* perspective.

As the theories became more complex, the models more sophisticated, and the techniques more intricate, my enthusiasm continued to wane. This was the antithesis of what I had experienced in my brief encounter with Virginia Satir. The "system" she used as a framework for her work had become the focus of the enterprise. Her curiosity and concern for individuals had been replaced by a detached obsession with the "model." And her impressive interpersonal skills had been translated into repetitive "communication" techniques. Whenever I had the opportunity to observe the leading figures in action, I invariably came away disheartened. With few exceptions, that wonderful opening up of energy generated by people finding and sharing their own self-expressions was sadly lacking. And the kids who had always been at the center of my concern and curiosity were somehow lost in the shuffle.

Like most ideas that are intuitively compelling and seemingly self-evident, the proposition that family intervention offers the greatest potential for change remains largely unsubstantiated. This does not mean that those of us who work with individual children should forget about the child's family. We do not need masses of research evidence to tell us that our most formative learning takes place through our earliest relational experiences or that our sense of Self emerges through interaction with those who are most significant–parents, siblings, or surrogates. Nor should we challenge those professionals who consider the family as their "client" on the grounds that the effects of their "interventions" are equivocal. Empirically speaking the evidence is no more or less convincing than anything to be found in the field of psychotherapy or child and youth care, for that matter. In my judgment, this will always be the case. My alternative proposition is that theories, methods, and techniques do not change lives or bring about personal growth. Change, growth, or transformation occurs only when people create the conditions in which responsible self-expression becomes possible, and this they must do for themselves, with or without professional assistance. So if we are looking for measures of success, it is time to reshape our research designs, redefine our objectives, and examine a completely different set of variables.

In articulating a child and youth care perspective on the family, we should not begin with the assumption that our focus on the immediate and developmental needs of the individual child is essentially inadequate or functionally misdirected. In particular, we should not be intimidated by those purveyors of "systems theory" who argue that the attention given to the "problems" of one member of the family will reinforce the belief that he or she is the one who needs to change. Certainly this is a possibility to be considered but, when all is said and done, a child is more than a family member and needs to be acknowledged as a separate and unique human being in his or her own right. As with any brand of professional intervention, it is not so much a question of what is done as how it is done–and by whom.

The challenge is to create a child and youth care perspective on families that does not lose sight of the primary focus on the individual child, and I do not believe this can be achieved by simply tacking on a few ideas borrowed from other professions. Given my stance that lasting change takes place from the *inside-out*, I have long maintained that our essential concern should be with the subjective experience of the child (Fewster, 1990). A fundamental aspect of that world is the family as it is experienced and understood by the individual child. My curiosity, then, is about the family as a subjective reality that is constructed collectively and experienced individually. If I look through the eyes of the child, I find myself peering into a unique relational configuration that can never be understood through its observable characteristics. In other words, I see the family in much the same way as I see the individual.

The thoughts presented in this paper are intended to offer only a possible point of departure. You will find no definitive theories, no claims of "truth," and no cook-book prescriptions. That is how it should be. If we are to create a child and youth care approach to families, then we must remain true to the experiential and exploratory nature of this profession. There are places, particularly in the discussion on systems theory, where the ideas may seem far removed from the everyday world of child and youth care. I invite you to press on regardless. If we are to continue to develop as a profession, it is important to ensure that we are not operating in a perceptual, cognitive, or experiential vacuum. To draw from other cultures does not contaminate the integrity of our own and to listen to what others have to say does not make us a slave to their ideas.

THE ELUSIVE FAMILY

You can take the child out of the family but you can never take the family out of the child. This may sound like a cliché, but for anyone who works with young people (or adults, for that matter), it is a plain and simple truth. Even where children have been physically separated from their family of origin since infancy, their earliest experiences of being with significant others continue to live on, forming a blue print for all future relationships. According to the most recent research in pre- and perinatal psychology, this process of learning actually begins well before birth as the developing fetus seeks to create relationships with mother and those who are closest to her (e.g., Chamberlain, 1999; Noble, 1993; Verny, 1981). Such early influences are profound and pervasive, but since they exist within the subjective experience of the individual, they can never be fully grasped from the outside, no matter how brilliant or intuitive the observer might be.

By the same token, competent professionals understand that when they work with individuals they are also working with that person's family in one way or another. Whatever issues or problems are being addressed are rooted somewhere in family relationships, and all change must ultimately come to terms with what was first learned in this context. Again, this is not the family as defined and assessed by outside observers but the unique configuration of significant relationships embedded within the conscious and unconscious world of each individual family member. Once this perspective is fully understood and incorporated into practice, it might be argued that all therapy is family therapy.

Given their concern for the well-being of individual children, child and youth care professionals may come to view families as alien or even hostile arrangements that contribute to the current difficulties and continue to undermine the child's progress–an attitude that can easily turn into objectification and blame. But this judgmental and moralistic stance not only ignores crucial information, it dismisses a fundamental aspect of the young person's world. Families are neither good nor bad. To some extent they all serve to meet the needs of their members and, in some ways, they are all neglectful and injurious. The task of the practitioner is not to judge–or even analyze–what they see but to remain curious about the child's experience life on the inside.

Child and youth care practitioners who do attempt to consider the family from the outside may find themselves overwhelmed by the prospect of intervening in this confusing and complex arena. To complicate matters even further, many of their clients have moved from the family of origin into alternative or surrogate arrangements that are tenuous or transitory. The worlds of these children are constructed from an intricate network of relationships, past and present, that can only be fleshed out through the most careful and sensitive professional approaches. Yet spurred on by their own ambitions and encouraged by those who advocate "systemic," "contextual," or "ecological" perspectives, misguided practitioners may come to believe that it is their task to change these conditions in the best interests of the child. But, as many community social workers have discovered to their dismay, any form of tinkering or heavy-handed intervention that fails to consider the child's sense of family can result in unforeseen and even tragic outcomes.

Given the confusion, it is hardly surprising that the profession of child and youth care has remained tentative in its attitude toward working with families and that individual practitioners tend to restrict their involvement to specific strategies such as parent training or child advocacy. Yet child and youth care will never address the needs of young people effectively until it finds a way to incorporate the family within its professional parameters. This means the creation of a clearly defined perspective that can be translated into effective child and youth care training and practice. The task may not be as difficult as it might appear once the underlying principles have been established. To this end, I have already articulated one firm foundational premise that fits for me–*the primary concern of the practitioner is with the subjective experience of the child or young person.*

THE FAMILY AS A "COMPLEX" SYSTEM

"Strategic" family therapists generally view the family as a system that can be modified through external intervention. For the uninitiated, this can be an intimidating stance involving complex theories, recurring dynamics, and intricate interventions. But those who are overawed by such sophisticated designs may wish to consider that all relationships are actually systemic, from the arrangement of subatomic particles and galaxies to the relationship between one adult and one child. In its original form, the discovery of how systems operate does not belong to psychology but to physics. As such, the principles and terminology of systems theory may seem remote from the more popular theories of child and youth care, but the basics are relatively straightforward and certainly worthy of our consideration.

To simplify the task, we might begin with the assumption that all systems fall into one of two broad categories. *Simple* systems, drawn from Newtonian principles, are those that operate mechanically and predictably with each part playing a constant role in the functioning of the whole, much like a wind-up clock or car engine. When they are operating efficiently, simple systems move toward a state of optimal balance or homeostasis that can be enhanced through external manipulation or fine tuning. *Complex* or emergent systems, drawn from the exciting world of quantum physics (e.g., Waldrop, 1992) are those in which each part possesses the ability to inform every other part through the expression of its own unique potential. Through the sharing of this information, all parts operate together to create a collective and dynamic whole. As an emerging entity, the experience of the whole, in turn, informs and influences the parts to produce a system that has its own specific purpose and its own internal integrity. Such systems, if they remain healthy, are constantly moving toward increased growth and complexity. Theoretically, their potential is infinite. The key to growth is the availability of new and accurate "information" that can be accessed and assimilated by all parts and at all levels. Some of this information is generated internally, and some is drawn from the outside, the broader context in which the particular system operates. Deficits or distortions from either source limit the system's developmental possibilities.

Both types of systems rely upon the same universal force: energy. In general, the simple system draws its energy from the outside. A clock works when it is wound-up or energized by electricity, and a car engine runs on the energy stored within its fossil fuels. While all energy is drawn from a single universal source, complex systems are constantly generating their own energetic requirements through their internal dynamic activity. In both cases, the system will fail to operate effectively if the energetic flow is disrupted or blocked and will simply close down if the energy is withdrawn. By the same token, if the system is to maintain its overall purpose and internal integrity, the energy of the parts and the whole must be contained within specific parameters or *boundaries*.

The essential difference between these two systemic arrangements is absolutely critical for anyone who chooses to apply systems theory to the field of human life and human relations. Traditionally, psychologists have relied upon a simple systems model to develop their own brands of theory and methodology. For this reason, their formulations have remained essentially mechanistic. But if we begin with the proposition that all relational systems involving human motivation and consciousness are potentially complex arrangements that, given the right conditions, are capable of infinite growth and development, the picture changes dramatically. Remember Virginia Satir?

In human relationships, the right conditions are those in which each Self (a complex system in its own right) is free to express its full potential within the experience of the whole. Consciousness, or awareness, implies that the necessary external and internal information is shared and assimilated effectively. This is referred to as an "open" system–one in which the parts and the whole operate from the same unrestricted informational base. Such an ideal is difficult to imagine in the imperfect world of human relationships, but that is not the point. The important question is a matter of degree and whether the system is moving toward higher levels of openness and growth or toward closure and atrophy. Referring back to an earlier point, this can only be known through the subjective experience of those who are directly involved in the system.

Viewed from this perspective, the human family offers an interesting case in point. A cynic might argue that the traditional family is essentially a closed system, more concerned with maintaining the distribution of power than the open sharing of information. To the degree that it operates as a role-based configuration, individuals are restricted in their ability to express their own unique qualities and the energy becomes stifled or blocked. Since families are often locked into social and cultural prescriptions, information from the outside is strictly limited and systematically controlled. Under such conditions, the family may appear more like a simple mechanistic system, incapable of offering growth and development in whole or in part. Unfortunately, this is a state of affairs that is often cherished in the name of family values.

While we all know families that operate this way (perhaps even our own), most of us are also aware of families that maintain high levels of openness and energy without sacrificing their essential structure or purpose. Children who grow up in such families are encouraged to bring themselves fully into the collective picture, each making his or her own unique contribution to the whole. Everybody has a place that carries specific responsibilities, yet the system remains responsive to new information, and every member has room to grow and the freedom to express themselves in their own way. Within the system, individual boundaries are respected and, within the broader context, the family is open to new information without sacrificing its sense of integrity. Such families are never ideal or perfect; they are simply personal environments in which new learning is an ever present and cherished possibility–creative and complex systems.

THE SIMPLE SIDE OF COMPLEXITY

From a systems perspective, then, the key to family (and personal) growth can be viewed as a shift toward increasing levels of complexity. While traditional theorists and practitioners might argue that this calls for strategic interventions into the system as a whole, change from the inside will occur as individual members express their own unique perspectives and potentials. If the system happens to be closed, such contributions will be resisted and, if that individual happens to be a child, the chances are that the internal power structures will move quickly and effectively to combat the challenge, in some cases rejecting the child in the process.

In such circumstances, the practitioner is confronted with an interesting dilemma. Within the professional relationship (a system in itself), he or she may invite the child to bring the Self forward while knowing that any changes in awareness or expression could pose a significant internal threat to the constitution of the family as a whole. Obviously, it would be unreasonable and potentially injurious to burden a child with the responsibility of changing his or her family from the inside. On the other hand, any attempt to impose limits on the child's growth to control for this possibility would be manipulative and blatantly unethical. In addition, the practitioner's personal beliefs and values about how the family *should* function can compound the predicament. A favorable evaluation from the outside might serve to reinforce the existing order, while any challenge may be perceived as an external threat and a signal for the family to close ranks.

One option might be to set all personal beliefs aside and settle for the widely accepted principle of parental authority. But from this position, child and youth care professionals can easily relinquish their primary commitment to the child in order to bring the troublesome youngster into line with parental expectations. The specific dangers inherent in such an alliance are obvious but, in the most general sense, the practitioner becomes an external agent serving the existing power structure. Another possibility might be to shift the focus from child development to some form of parent training. Unless the parents are drawn into personal therapy, such intervention generally takes the form of external prescriptions designed to influence specific behavioral patterns rather than attend to the more profound issues of personal development and interpersonal growth.

Alternatively, changes brought about through the expression of individual Selves challenge others to respond at the same level. Systemically speaking, the reasons, the resources, and the readiness for change are all contained within the family. While additional information might be made available from outside, it is the family as a whole that must make its own adjustments in its own way, preserving its own inherent sense of boundary and integrity in the process. In this, professionals must constantly remind themselves that the potential for change lies within and among the members of the family; only the family can come to know how the system operates and how it might work more effectively and creatively for their mutual benefit. In this sense, again, working with a family is really no different than working with an individual.

While practitioners who work with individual children will never come to know the full reality of life within the family any more than they can come to know the subjective world of an individual, they can still maintain a systemic perspective. Through their curiosity about the child's experience they create opportunities for mutual exploration and the consideration of options. In this way, they can begin to understand what contextual factors might facilitate or inhibit the youngster's growth and development. In particular, they can become increasingly aware of family responses to whatever changes the child might make. Again, this is not about the actual or observable responses of family members. What really matters is *how the child experiences them for his or her place in the family*. What may appear to be a critical issue from the outside may have little or no consequence for the child, while a seemingly innocuous parental gesture might arouse the child's most deeply rooted fears of rejection and abandonment.

Within the safety of their relationship, the practitioner may encourage the child to express the Self, explore potentials, and take risks that would not be considered possible within the context of the family. At the same time, the systemically aware professional understands that, if the child is to learn and grow from such experiences, the support of the family will be essential. He or she will also understand how families that come to appreciate the unique potential of each individual member create an environment that supports the well-being and growth of the whole. In this sense, the child who is exploring his or her own potential outside the family context can be a catalyst for systemic change but, as with all challenges to the Self, the process is never a stroll in the park. For the practitioner, working with a child through this process demands considerable skill and sensitivity–the essential attributes of a professional.

First and foremost, the practitioner must always keep the young person as the focal point of attention. The child's subjective experience is the critical reference point for change and the window through which the practitioner can best understand what might be taking place beneath the presented attitudes and observable behavior of the family. While the picture might never be clear or definitive, the enlightened professional always knows that, when it comes to change, the family has the capacity and the resources to create its own developmental pathway. The most important issue is that individual *boundaries* be articulated and respected. Without clear and effective personal boundaries, it is impossible for family members to own and express their personal experiences. Unfortunately, it is not possible to deal adequately with this topic within the present discussion, but a few words of clarification might be helpful.

In this context, the term "boundary" is not about prescribed roles, rules, and regulations; it refers to the energetic, cognitive, emotional, and behavioral parameters of the Self (Rand and Fewster, 1997; Rosenberg and Kitean-Morse, 1996). As such, a boundary contains the subjective experience of the Self and makes it possible for such information to be shared in a clear and self-responsible way. On the other side, people who are secure in their personal boundaries are able to listen to others without imposing their own experiences or agendas in the process. In other words, they are fully aware of where they end and others begin. This is a necessary condition for all effective relationships and for any form of interpersonal work. As such, professionals who choose to work from the subjective experience of their clients must be highly skilled in encouraging others to become aware of their own boundaries and how to establish them in relationships. But this is only possible if practitioners are secure in their own sense of boundary and, in most cases, this requires considerable personal work. Apart from understanding and respecting the boundaries of individuals, they should also be aware that families–as interpersonal systems–have their own boundaries that need to be acknowledged and respected. Practitioners who are unaware of other people's boundaries are clumsy, intrusive, and potentially injurious to those they seek to help.

Given that effective boundaries are in place, it is possible to be naively curious about a child's experience of life in his or her family without imposing judgements or unwarranted interpretations from the outside. In this way, the practitioner can become an effective listener, a mirror through which the young person can begin to recognize his or her unique experiences and potentials. Through this process, the Self is revealed and acknowledged and, in the presence of a skilled collaborator, the Self will draw from its own resources, enabling the individual to return to the pathway of self-directed and self-responsible growth. But the matter of whether such changes will meet with resistance or promote growth within the family still needs to be addressed.

For growth to occur, the young person must be willing and able to introduce this new information into the family system in a clear, respectful, and responsible manner. Once the necessary awareness, confidence, and skills have been developed through working with the practitioner, the child will probably need considerable support and validation in taking this next critical step. On the other side, members of the family–particularly the parents–must be prepared to listen without sensing that their personal authority or the integrity of their family is at risk. In all of this the role of the professional remains delicately balanced. If he or she is seen as an advocate for the child, the doors may remain firmly closed, while a stance of detached neutrality might serve to confirm that whatever the child has to say is essentially irrelevant or insignificant. Alternatively, any apparent alliance with the parents is likely to be perceived by the child as an act of abandonment or betrayal and a confirmation of the status quo by other members of the family.

Even for the most skilled and seasoned practitioner, this involves an act of faith–an understanding that lasting change will only occur when both the child and the family are able to draw upon their own internal resources. The essential role of the professional is to assist in creating conditions in which the experience of the child will be perceived as information that might add to rather than detract from the well-being of the family. Creating a climate of respect and safety through the articulation of boundaries is always the first step and, in this, the practitioner must be absolutely clear in establishing his or her place in the scheme of things. Theoretically, the task is quite straightforward–to serve as a competent and concerned external presence while members of the family generate and assimilate new information through sharing their thoughts, feelings, and experiences *with each other.*

In practice, however, this is no simple matter. In many cases, the child's need for an advocate, the family's need for an authority or arbitrator, and the practitioner's need to make something happen can combine to direct the flow of communication outside the system. In order to create an effective place on the outside, the boundary between the professional and the family must be particularly clear and rigorously maintained. All ideas about being an expert, a problem solver, or an advocate must be shelved to make way for the only expertise that really matters: the ability to stay with the process while teaching and modeling boundaries, inviting others to come forward, seeking clarification, and encouraging interpersonal feedback. Since all families are unique and practitioners vary in their range of skills and options, there is no standard or clear-cut way of achieving this. In some cases it might be necessary or desirable to begin work with the young person and one other family member, preferably a parent. Or it may be an option to work with the family as a whole.

Given all of the potential distractions, child and youth care professionals who attempt to assume a broad systemic perspective must find ways to maintain their focus on the subjective experience of the child. This is always home base, the nexus for the work, and the defining principle of the profession. Despite all I have said thus far, it would be naïve to assume that the child or any family member, for that matter, is fully aware of that experience and is ready to share his or her analysis with some curious bystander. Inviting the child to explore this inner world and finding ways of communicating whatever is discovered is the essence of the child and youth care relationship. While some people, like Virginia Satir, seem to have an inherent ability to generate trust and safety from the outset, for most of us the development of such relationships is a sensitive and gradual process. To a large extent, the mutual learning that takes place between the young person and the practitioner becomes the model for the exploration for what is taking place in the family and for relationships in general.

From any perspective, configurations of relational influences within families are complex and far reaching. Within the subjective personal and interpersonal world of any given family, the picture can be even more obscure and perplexing. At the beginning of this paper, I mentioned how pre- and perinatal researchers have shown that specific relational themes and patterns are established well before birth but, to take one more step back, it is clear that they actually begin before conception, embedded in the intergenerational history of the family. By becoming aware of these patterns and themes it is possible to create a framework in which the ubiquitous and often chaotic world of each individual can be more clearly seen and understood. For this reason, many family therapists invite their clients to construct a family map or genealogy that looks back two or three generations. While this exercise is undoubtedly valuable, the problem is that the typical genealogy is constructed from stories or facts passed from one family member to another. As such, the finished product is essentially detached from the subjective experience of the individual, although he or she may have some thoughts and feelings about whatever is shared or documented.

To address this problem, psychotherapist Jack Rosenberg (Rosenberg, Rand, & Asay, 1985; Rosenberg & Kitaen-Morse, 1996) developed an investigative tool that examines relational patterns across generations *from the perspective of the client.* Referred to as the "primary scenario," this method calls upon the expertise of the practitioner in assisting the client to flesh out what it means and how it feels to be part of his or her particular family from the earliest memories to the present moment in time. In other words, the family history becomes incorporated into the immediate experience of the client. Since this process incorporates and exemplifies many of the skills necessary for professionals working from the subjective experience of their clients, it would be ideal to review this method in detail. Unfortunately, such an analysis lies beyond the scope of this paper but, if working from the inside-out is to become a legitimate and effective principle of professional child and youth care practice, then we are challenged by Rosenberg's example to create and refine methods appropriate to the task. As things stand, they are few and far between.

A POINT OF DEPARTURE

To return to the task of articulating a child and youth care orientation of work with families, I am suggesting that, given the focus on the subjective world of the child, the methods we create should always respect and respond to that translucent reality. To provide some structure for this exercise, it might be useful to begin with a set of questions that seem to be relevant, based upon our existing levels of understanding and our current areas of curiosity. The questions proposed in this section make sense to me based upon my own experience in working with children. They are not intended to represent an "assessment" in any shape or form; they are simply designed to offer possible avenues of enquiry. While they all have some general theoretical significance, they should be quickly dismissed or modified if they are seen to be irrelevant to the subjective or inter-

personal world of the child. As you go through them you will probably think of
questions that should be added; please do so.

THE CHILD'S EXPERIENCE OF THE FAMILY AS A WHOLE

What are the basic rules and expectations for membership in this family?
Who actually qualifies for membership? (siblings, aunts, uncles, lodgers, etc.)
Who has the power in this family? How is that power distributed or shared?
How are feelings expressed in this family? (affection, anger, fear, etc.)
How does this family relate to the world? (extended family, community, etc.)
Is this family a safe place to be?
Who most represents the values and attitudes of this family?
Who is responsible for instilling these values and attitudes?
What does the pattern of attachments look like?
What happens when this family faces a crisis?
What does it mean to have fun in this family?
What does it mean to be a female in this family?
What does it mean to be a male in this family?
Is there excessive use of drugs or alcohol in this family?
Do people keep their promises in this family?
Is there physical affection in this family?
How is sexuality expressed in this family?
Are there secrets in this family?
Does the child have his/her own place in this family?
How are conflicts dealt with/resolved in this family?

THE CHILD'S RELATIONAL EXPERIENCE

Does the child feel loved and wanted? How? By whom? For what?
Who does the child feel closest to? Why?
What is the nature of this bond?
What does the child have to do to maintain this relationship?
What is the child's relationship to mother?
What is the child's relationship to the other parent? (if applicable)
Who does the child most want to please?
What is the child's relationship to other siblings? (if applicable)
Who does the child most admire/respect?
Does the child feel seen and heard? By whom?
Who would the child most like to be like? Why?
Who does the child most like to be with? Why?

Who is the child most likely to share his/her troubles with? Why?
Are the child's accomplishments recognized? By whom?
Does the child feel important/special to others?
How is the child disciplined? By whom? For what?
Does the child feel free to express his/her sexuality?
Does the child feel punished? By whom? For what?
Does this child feel responsible for the happiness of others? (parents, siblings, etc.)
Is the child physically, emotionally, or sexually abused? By whom?

SUMMARILY YOURS...

Most professionals view the family as a tangible reality: an observable relational context in which people learn about themselves, each other, and the world in which they live. For these practitioners, working with the family means involving the members in some process designed to bring about attitudinal and behavioral changes in the way people respond and relate to each other. In the preceding pages, I have suggested that child and youth care professionals might consider the family in a different way: as a fundamental and on-going aspect of subjective experience. From this perspective, the family experience emerges as a unique personal reality that constantly influences the individual's sense of Self and the development of relationships throughout the life-span. Working from the *inside-out*, the task of the practitioner is to invite the client to become aware of this inner reality, to consider options that promote personal development, and to draw upon personal resources to make the choices that express each individual's sense of Self.

In my opinion and experience, this is an approach that is ideally suited to child and youth care practice. It allows the practitioner to be unquestionably child-centered without discounting the context in which the young person lives. It extrapolates the skills that have become synonymous with this profession and draws us away from the agendas of those who would measure success in terms of obedience and conformity. At the broadest level it reflects values that invite us to explore the full experience of what it means to be human, to be all that we are, and to find new ways of being together in a self-responsible and loving way. Imagine that.

REFERENCES

Chamberlain, D. (1999). Life in the womb: Dangers and opportunities. *Journal of Prenatal and Perinatal Psychology and Health, 14*(1-2), 31-45.
Fewster, G. (1990). *Being in child care: A journey into self.* New York: The Haworth Press, Inc.
Fewster, G. (1992). Ask Charlotte. *Journal of Child and Youth Care, 7*(3), 91-95.
Noble, E. (1993). *Primal connections.* New York: Simon and Schuster, Inc.

Rand, M., & Fewster, G. (1997). Self, boundaries and containment: Integrative body psychotherapy. In C. Caldwell (Ed.), *Getting in touch: The guide to new body-centered therapies* (pp. 71-89). Illinois: Quest Books.

Rosenberg, J., & Kitaen-Morse, B. (1996). *The intimate couple.* Atlanta: Turner Publishing, Inc.

Rosenberg, J., Rand, M., & Asay, D. (1985). *Body, self and soul: Sustaining integration.* Atlanta: Humanics.

Verny, T. (1981). *The secret life of the unborn child.* New York. Delacorte.

Waldrop, M. (1992). *Complexity: The emerging science at the edge of order and chaos.* New York: Simon and Schuster.

Guidelines in Child and Youth
Care Family Work:
A Case Story

Grant Charles
Holly Charles

SUMMARY. There are many paths that can be taken with the families we encounter in our work. It is this richness in options that can make the child and youth care approach so powerful. However, amongst each potential path there are a number of common guideposts that serve as markers for our interactions with families. These guiding principles are described through the use of examples from a family in a program for teens who are parenting. *[Article copies available for a fee from The Haworth Document Delivery Service: 1-800-HAWORTH. E-mail address: <docdelivery@haworthpress.com> Website: <http://www.HaworthPress.com> © 2003 by The Haworth Press, Inc. All rights reserved.]*

KEYWORDS. Youthwork with families, youth care work, social work with families, family-centered residential care, child and youth care, family services, family support, parent education, residential care work and families

We do not believe there is just one avenue of intervention when taking a child and youth care approach to working with families. Instead, we would like

---

Grant Charles is affiliated with the University of British Columbia. Holly Charles is affiliated with Catholic Family Services, Calgary, Alberta.

[Haworth co-indexing entry note]: "Guidelines in Child and Youth Care Family Work: A Case Story." Charles, Grant, and Holly Charles. Co-published simultaneously in *Child & Youth Services* (The Haworth Press, Inc.) Vol. 25, No. 1/2, 2003, pp. 95-115; and: *A Child and Youth Care Approach to Working with Families* (ed: Thom Garfat) The Haworth Press, Inc., 2003, pp. 95-115. Single or multiple copies of this article are available for a fee from The Haworth Document Delivery Service [1-800-HAWORTH, 9:00 a.m. - 5:00 p.m. (EST). E-mail address: docdelivery@haworthpress.com].

to suggest that there are many paths that can be taken on a daily basis with the families we encounter. It is this richness in options that makes the child and youth care approach so powerful. We do believe that amongst these potential paths there are a number of common guideposts for our interactions with families. This article will outline these guiding principles through the use of examples from the experiences the second author has had working with a young woman, Jane, and her son, Andrew, in a program for teens who parent as well as with Jane's mother and father.

The Louise Dean Program is a joint partnership between Calgary Catholic Family Services, the Calgary Board of Education, and the Calgary Health Region. The partnership has been in place for almost thirty years and is unique in both its longevity and approach. Catholic Family Services provides on-site and outreach intervention and support programs. The Calgary Board of Education provides on-site educational services, and the Calgary Regional Health provides on-site prenatal and postnatal health services. In addition, the Louise Dean Program works in partnership with a number of other local service providers. The result is that a full spectrum of services is offered to what in many jurisdictions is an often-underserved population. The program receives funding from the Province of Alberta, the city of Calgary, Health Canada, and a number of private donors. While this chapter will focus primarily on the family support work of the program run by Catholic Family Services, it is important to note that the success of each of the partner component parts of the program is dependent upon the assistance and cooperation of the other partners. In a true systemic manner, the effectiveness of the program as a whole is greater and more powerful than the impact the individual partners would have if they were to offer stand-alone services.

The mandate of the Catholic Family Services portion of the Louise Dean Program is to support pregnant or parenting adolescents and youth in creating a stable family environment by reducing the risks commonly associated with clients in this age group. The program offers counselling services to individuals, couples, and families, and provides teaching and mentoring services for young mothers through specialized learning centers. The community outreach program also provides in-home early childhood education to parenting teens and their children as well as in-home support of a more involved nature for the specific needs of the young people.

The focus of these interventions is improving the capacity of the young people in family, life, school, and community situations while reducing environmental risks. Success for the program is defined as stable functioning in several domains for both mother and child, a process that, we have learned, takes a minimum of eighteen months. A variety of parent/child measurement tools are used to determine that stability. For example, we look at finances, education, housing, personal support, and social supports as areas that require attention in order for a young mom to be ready emotionally and physically to attend to the needs of her child. We also look at risk factors for parenting, such as poor lifestyle choices and physical and/or mental health risks, to mitigate the need for child protection services. The bottom line for front-line workers is to help a young mom be the best mother possible.

Due to their young age, the young women and young fathers– when they are involved–have developmental needs, unlike new families established by people in their twenties or later, that mean they are still children and yet, because of their circumstances, they are also adults. This happens to all of us in some way or another but they have to master a series of developmental tasks in a parallel process rather than in the more usual sequential manner that most of us experience.

In this article we will look at a number of the principles of a child and youth care approach when working with families, using for illustration the relationship one of the authors has had with a young client of the program over several years. Jane, the young woman, is now 19 years old. She is the mother of a three-year-old son. She has been involved with the program in one fashion or another for four years. Please note that her name and some of the details of her story have been changed.

JANE'S STORY

Jane was referred to the school program at the Louise Dean Centre because of her pregnancy. She had previously been attending a school program for behavior-disordered youth, and the pregnancy presented safety concerns in that school. Jane's parents agreed with the school change and, although not happy about the pregnancy, they supported their daughter's decision to carry the pregnancy to term and would work out the parenting issues as time went by. It became apparent that Jane and her family have had many issues to deal with over several years. The history suggests that a number of behavioral and academic concerns arose in early elementary school and, despite assessments and family involvement, little success was sustained. As Jane approached adolescence, her behaviors became more problematic for the family, and they turned to child protection services for help. Unfortunately for this family, their involvement with child protection services did not go well. Jane's behaviors escalated (she was hospitalized for a suicide attempt), and the family was forced to consider residential care. The family believes that in this program Jane was subjected to knowledge and experience that constituted abuse and fought to have her return to the home with therapeutic supports in place. The family entered into family coun selling, couples counselling, and Jane went to individual counselling. They also welcomed a family support worker into the home to assist with family routines. When Jane came to the Louise Dean Centre her family had been involved with the helping professions for at least three years and were seeing little success. Jane's father was the primary caregiver for the family. He worked full time and managed the household of six. Jane's mother worked part time and was in therapy for depression and issues of childhood abuse. Jane's siblings were all in school and attending regularly, although two of the boys had behavioral problems and poor grades.

In consultation with Jane's team at the Louise Dean Centre, a strategy to engage Jane in the school milieu of the school was established as our primary goal. She needed to see our environment as safe with normal expectations for a 15-year-old high school student. Our goal was to provide Jane with a setting in which she could achieve her academic goals, make the best decision possible regarding parenting choices for herself and her family, and to engage her in a therapeutic relationship that did not duplicate her relationships with her "therapists." An approach of building the relationship through trust and non-hierarchical interactions was chosen and proved to be successful.

While there was no doubt that this young women was experiencing many struggles in her life, we believed that she had the right to the same experiences that other people her age could expect. Our interactions with her would not be focused solely upon her presenting problems but as much or more so upon her person and her developmental needs. Effective and respectful practice requires that presenting problems are seen as manifestations of human pain and do not constitute the whole person (Kottler, 1991; Pearce & Pezzot-Pearce, 1997).

SETTING THE STAGE

Our first interactions with our clients do not always go the way we would ideally like, of course. What then becomes important is to look past the obvious to what is being expressed behind it, and it is often a hurt and a pain masked by anger and rejection.

I met Jane for the first time at a school conference. She was being transferred to our program from a treatment setting, because the program staff felt that she was not safe vis-à-vis the pregnancy. Further, she was sullen, angry, and disrespectful to her father. She indicated through body language and facial expressions that this new program "sucked" and in no way was she buying into it! She stated that she would attend but not to expect anything from her.

Many of our clients, like Jane, have not had positive experiences with the helping system. They tend to be distrustful of us and remain skeptical of what the system has to offer them (Fox, 1994; Philion, 2002).

> Jane did not see any reason to change. She was well versed by this time in therapeutic talk and was a master at persuasion and manipulation of adults and her peers. Her control needs were huge! She was bright and saw through anyone's attempts to intervene without her consent. If the consequence was in her favor, Jane would go along with such interventions until they interfered in some way with what she wanted, and then she would resist. For example, child protection services were part of her life for a period of time, and she gladly accepted the condition of engaging with a youth worker they imposed on her, because it meant a ride to school every morning, whereas the condition to see a mental health therapist weekly was met but with a great deal of passive resistance and, as a result, little change occurred.

Despite the emphasis upon normalizing her experiences, one cannot in practice ignore the issues in her life. However, the best way to deal with the issues is to take a longer-term view of how change will occur (Garfat, 1998). Successes big or small have to be celebrated both because of the meaning they have to Jane in the present but also because of what it will mean in the future.

> Jane struggled in many areas of daily life. She had significant learning problems, life threatening health concerns, and a family life that has been chaotic and was ambivalent around parenting when under stress. Any change in these domains influenced the others, whether the change was positive or negative. When Jane had success at school, her health conditions stabilized, and she was better able to enjoy her child.

By the time many of our clients have come to us, they are quite jaded by their experiences. They are particularly upset about having to tell their stories time and time again as if telling the story itself is somehow healing (Charles, 1996). Jane wanted to have control over her story in a way that she never had control of her past.

> Jane did not arrive at our door untouched by life's unsavoury aspects. She proclaimed she'd been in therapy since she was 12 and it hadn't done a thing for her! Her story was often contradictory and unfinished, and early on in the relationship I made the decision in cooperation with her that the past belonged to her, and she could share it with me if needed. She was always worried that people would judge her based upon her behavior and not see that she was making efforts to make changes in her life. There was the reality that her past issues did influence her current behavior and that our work together would focus upon learning to make more positive choices. In this way, we could be pre-emptive and begin to change the patterns of impulsivity.

Trust is the foundation of any relationship (Austin & Halpin, 1989; Coady, 1993; Garfat, 1998; Ross & Hoeltke, 1987). Without it, long-term change is unlikely to occur. However, given that many of our clients have no reason to trust anyone–least of all someone who they perceive to have power over them as many helpers do–trust can take a long time to develop. Even then it is often quite fragile.

> Trust was and continues to be the thread that allows Jane to establish relationships with others. Gaining her trust was a year-long process of just being present. It was important to establish the boundaries of the relationship that safeguarded my professional role without the staid structure of the professional relationship. I needed also to be aware of the impact that breaking trust, even in the smallest incident, would have on our relationship.

It is also important to be respectful of the distance our clients occasionally need from us (Charles, 1996). Respecting their desire to have control of the relationship in this manner reaps long-term benefits.

> Jane has worked with me for four years and the frequency and intensity of the work has been varied as has the honesty and commitment within the relationship. There was a pattern to the ebb and flow early on: to share her successes and hide her poor choices. Now Jane is able to share the decisions she makes.

Many of the people we work with need an anchor in their lives (Garfat, 1998; Pearce & Pezzot-Pearce, 1997). They need something they can grab onto and go with over time. They need to have a place where they can experience a sense of mastery over their lives.

For Jane, it is education. If she succeeds at school, she succeeds at life. Completing high school heralds the rest of her life. Jane came to me through a school program, and she remains in school programs even though there have been times over the four years when withdrawing from school would have reduced the stress in her life. School provides a safety net for this young person: a place to go, a place for friendships, a place of unconditional regard. Jane has been lucky to have support people in place who have assisted her in maintaining her school status.

THE CONTEXT

Being aware of the developmental level of the client along with the corresponding tasks for them to complete is an important first step in engagement. However, understanding this developmental process is not as simple or as straightforward as it seems in the textbooks.

As with all the young women in our program, Jane was a child having a child. There are complicating developmental issues when teens have children. While it is the teen's job to differentiate themselves from their family, develop a self-identity and prepare for emancipation, the psychological tasks of pregnancy demand an acknowledgement of the responsibility for another and the reconnection with mothers through the shared experience of motherhood.

One of the ways to gain this sense of mastery is to break the tasks we have to accomplish into manageable portions. Clients need to have the opportunity to learn in a manner and at a pace that is respectful of everything else that is happening in their lives.

Jane could only deal with these developmental influences by compartmentalizing her roles, such as mother, student, daughter, and friend. For example, in the Louise Dean Centre the young moms are encouraged to visit the learning centres (child care) during the day to feed and assist generally with the care of their child. In doing this, they are provided one-on-one teaching from the child-care staff. Jane's style of utilizing this service was either to immerse herself in the learning center milieu and do a lot of parenting tasks at the expense of her classes, or she did not attend at all and immersed herself in her studies. The ability to balance both tasks was difficult and, over time, Jane saw use of the learning center as a break from parenting for at least six hours a day. During those hours she could concentrate on being a student and developing friends. She did school work only during the school hours, which led to incomplete courses.

Spending time with friends is important for adolescents, and Jane was no different in this need. However, for the teen mom, non-mom friends place expectations on the friendship that they are not able to meet. If she is not spending time with her child while in classes, the time for parenting is in the evenings, and this often interferes with the time to spend with friends. In Jane's case, she often left the evening parenting to her family while she spent time with friends. The reconnection with her mother never materialized due to ongoing conflict.

When Jane and I reviewed her parenting time, she could see she was compartmentalizing that role along with all the others. However, her ability to understand that she needed to strive for integration of her roles is not yet successful. This is evident when Jane chooses to place herself in a high-risk situation. She believes she is only harming herself because she has made sure that her child is being cared for by her family. She does not see the risk to herself as an individual having any bearing on how she will be perceived as a mother.

Child and youth care has a strong history of teamwork within the profession (Krueger, 1991) and with partners in the related helping fields. This teamwork directly assists our clients by increasing the range of help that can be offered. Teamwork helps us by supporting us in situations that are often hard to deal with on a regular basis.

Being an effective treatment team with a young person like Jane requires a level of teamwork not often found amongst agencies. Jane's community outreach worker, teacher, and mental health therapist all agreed that direct and frequent communication was essential to providing Jane with a consistent treatment plan. Therefore, we were able to be available for case conferencing and, with Jane's consent, also able to confer without her presence. This collegiality allowed the key support people in her life to construct fairly accurate details of the events that concerned her and also the events in which she was progressing. We were able to provide similar messages of intervention without undermining one another's work. As a treatment team we were able to draw support from each other when Jane would be going through a rough patch. We were also able to help each other maintain clear boundaries in our work with a young person who preferred to triangulate her support systems.

THE ISSUES

Change is a slow process for many of our clients (Charles, 1996). They take a few steps forward and a couple back. It is important that we help them take a big picture view of their accomplishments so that their slips are seen as only temporary. We also have to learn patience as they struggle to adapt new ways of living their lives.

Jane's biggest accomplishment has been to live a street and drug free life, and this achievement gives her hope that she will find the motivation in time to cease other non-desirable behaviors. Jane's early adolescent and acting-out behaviors were focused on the street and drug culture. She tells a story that is typical of many young women who have been sexually abused in their childhoods: initial acceptance on the street of risk-taking behaviors and identification with others based on similarity of backgrounds, vulnerability leading to a relationship with a man who treated her as special, and then the pattern of drug use and eventual prostitution. Jane's pregnancy took her away from the street and drug culture, because during her pregnancy she made the health of her child her first priority. It has been a struggle for her to maintain this attitude as a priority over the years when financial need and emotional pain has served as an excuse for Jane to return to drugs and prostitution for some weekends.

Despite these relapses, Jane believes that her life on the streets is over because each transgression was harder and harder to overcome and the risks inherent are no longer worth it.

Change can be painful for all of us. This is particularly the case if one is feeling overwhelmed and isolated. As helpers, one of our responsibilities is to be able to acknowledge this pain for our clients and not to minimize it. Another responsibility is to be there when we are needed. One example from our work with Jane illustrates these.

> Jane's confidence in herself was low. She was attending school daily but getting little accomplished there, yet she received from her teacher some of the emotional support she craved. The teacher and I had been in daily telephone contact with each other for updates on her coping skills and sharing ideas and techniques to keep Jane stable. There had been a build-up of suicidal ideation, depressed mood, and a decline in her normally cathartic letter writing. Suicidal risk assessment placed her at moderate risk, and the family was alerted to be more vigilant during the coming long holiday weekend. Just before the weekend, Jane called me from an unused office at the school. She was in tears–distraught and suicidal. I had no concern that she was in immediate danger, but I knew the school staff needed to find her while I kept her talking. Fortunately, the walls of the offices in my organization are very thin, and an astute colleague could hear the seriousness of my call; when I knocked on the wall, she came to my office door. I was able to pass a note to her to call the teacher at the school with the information that I had Jane on the line. The teacher found Jane in about 10 minutes and just listened at the door. I was able to contract with Jane to remain at the school and seek out her teacher, and I would go there immediately to help her develop a safe plan for herself and her child.

There are times when it is easier to fall back into previous ways of interacting to get one's needs met (Pearce & Pezzot-Pearce, 1997). At times like this it is critical for the practitioner to be understanding of the reasons for the regression while at the same time confronting the behavior. The success of the confrontation depends on the manner in which it is put forward and the level of trust that has developed between you and the client. It is critical that the confrontation is both straightforward and supportive.

> For example, Jane has many health problems and it remains unclear at this time how many of these are the result of self-harming behaviors. Regardless of the cause, she seeks and needs medical attention frequently. However, Jane does not disclose pertinent, important information. She is ashamed of and embarrassed by her conditions and explains only what is needed for the treatment she is seeking, even though she is very bright and would like a career in the helping professions. Moreover, she is keen on medical terminology and will look up diseases, disorders, and medications online in order to speak at an equal level with physicians. As you can imagine, this is not always a very successful strategy for Jane. Recently, she experienced the harsh reality of medical dishonesty. On a visit to emergency for abdominal pain, she was accused of drug seeking and underwent an examination without analgesics. Her emergency room physician took a brief look through her very thick file and dismissed her need as not requiring compassion and understanding

but rather rudeness, disrespect, and humiliation. When Jane was retelling the story to me, it was very difficult to be empathetic. Jane had faced a situation where she usually succeeded at getting her own way, and much of her responses resembled a two-year-old's temper tantrum. Because of our relationship, she allowed me to challenge her responses in this situation and also to take the physician's point of view. It was also an opportunity to reiterate with her the need to maintain a primary physician who could advocate for her in these circumstances. Jane saw the sense in this approach and we worked on a plan for her to suggest to her primary physician within the week. When I offered to attend her next doctor's appointment with her, she felt she could handle it on her own. I took this as a statement that she was not yet committed to having a witness to her interactions with her physician and left it at that.

Another task for helpers is to assist clients to learn to see the world in a different way in order to negotiate the demands of life. As part of this we need to help clients learn to advocate for themselves in such a way so as to produce the results they desire and that are in their best interests.

Jane came with her son to visit me today. She wanted to discuss strategies for getting child welfare off her back. Once again, because of her self-harming behavior, child welfare was called by program staff concerned about her ability to meet the emotional needs of her child. As she talked and became worked up about what her lawyer was going to do, I stopped her and asked to see the support agreement. As I read through each item and we discussed her progress in each area, it was clear that Jane was meeting the requirements of the agreement. When I commented that the agreement appeared to be written with the intent for her to be successful, her response was, "Yes but . . ." Having anyone tell her what to do and when always meets her opposition, even if that opposition leads to undesirable results for her. Yet we were able to discuss the two remaining conditions to be met and were able to spend our time and energy strategizing about how these conditions could be met successfully in comparison to wasting time and energy fighting the system. Compliance with these few conditions could finally document for the Child Welfare file that Jane is indeed a good parent to her son. She still needs to learn how to pick her battles.

This advocacy is a critical component of our work. Too often clients experience the negative aspects of the helping systems rather than the positive ones.

Clients like Jane experience daily disrespect from the systems intended to assist them, but this disrespect is not necessarily institutionalized. It still appears to be dependent upon the individual person Jane interacts with. It was therefore essential that Jane practice interacting with other people within other systems and therefore the systems in general and provide advocacy when required. She experienced disrespect in the health, law, social, and educational systems. For example, there appeared to be little regard for confidentiality in the health system, and Jane's health status was known to other people without the proper authorizations from Jane or her parents. She found that teachers spoke freely about her situation in front of other students without sensitivity. She found herself targeted by law enforcement whenever she was in a questionable area of the city even if no illegal behavior was observed. She also experienced rude and harsh treatment by the social and health systems in place to provide assistance. Learning to address these injustices was difficult for Jane. Her inclination was to "lip off" the offending person but she learned that calling into question their need to treat her so poorly was more often met with an acknowledgement that the interaction could be more respectful.

THE FAMILY

We have to learn to recognize strength even in seemingly unlikely places (Dolan, 1991). It is this ability to recognize strength when others would only see the negative aspects of life that helps clients get in touch with the many skills that they have but do not recognize.

The first time I went to Jane's parents' house I was driving slowly along the street looking at house numbers when I spotted a house with an unkempt appearance at odds with the neighbourhood. "Don't let that be Jane's house," I thought, but it was. The home was too small to house Jane, her son, her mom, dad and siblings. Mom and another sibling were cleaning the kitchen when I arrived. The amount of debris at broom's end was significant and not just a few crumbs from lunch. The house retained an odour of staleness and unwashed clothes. And yet, as she worked, Jane sang out in a beautiful voice. This struck me as paradoxical: A family with mental health troubles, marital strife, single parenthood, and a generally chaotic lifestyle still managed to produce moments of beauty.

There are times when the reality of the situations of our clients is beyond what we can help them overcome. We have to learn where we can have an impact and where at the present time it is not possible for our clients to get what they need.

Ideally, Jane and her son needed a home where re-parenting of Jane could have occurred and, subsequently, better and more consistent parenting of her own child. However, Jane remained in her parents' home and, at times, this felt like the best and worst place for her. It was the best place for Jane to be because of the parental and sibling support she received for parenting. Her child was never alone and was loved equally by other family members. It was the worst place for Jane to be because of the longstanding conflict with her mother that could never be resolved even though a great deal of other professional help was focused upon this relationship.

Regardless of their past history, it is possible to engage the members of families to help each other (Pennell & Burford, 1994; Walsh, 2002). The important thing is that our expectation of how they can help each other has to match their current ability to do so. Unrealistic expectations–either too much or too little–just serve to disengage an avenue of possible support.

In Jane's case, her mother has been peripheral to our involvement with Jane over the years due to her unstable mental health. This dynamic within the family has not been difficult to work with because of the availability of Jane's father for case conferences. Jane's mother has been responsive to retrieving Jane when she would fall ill in school or when her grandson needed attention. Her role in Jane's chaotic behaviors has been suspect but never substantiated. Jane describes a very poor relationship with her mother and prefers not to speak about her. When she is suicidal, Jane will make reference to the wish that she had a mother who cared about her like other people do. Her greatest fear is to be like her mother when she grows up.

Yet in the next breath, Jane would tell a story about something fun she did with her mother and siblings, and it usually involved receiving money or a gift of some sort. Her need to be accepted by her mother is so great that a gift could buy that belief for a short time. The relationship between Jane and her mother has been the focus of her traditional therapy and not of ours.

Over time, there were many small successes in Jane's life, and we have to learn to experience with our clients all of the steps they take towards a healthier life. Celebration of the small victories makes the occasional defeats easier to overcome.

In one case, a voice-mail message caught my attention. A young but clear voice said, "Hi. This is Andrew and my mommy and I went to the zoo today . . . we saw elephants and giraffes . . . I had popcorn . . . oh yeah . . . call my mom when you have a chance." In the background I could hear Jane whispering to her son about what to say. I listened three times to this voice mail. I could hear in their voices how much fun the two of them were having. These moments were few and far between in my relationship with Jane. Most interactions were problem-focused. But one of her strengths was the bond with her son, and that is what I heard and could reflect to her in our next conversation.

THE MEANING OF FAMILY

Clients have a number of different families. We should not allow ourselves to get caught in seeing family solely as biological. Family is what we make it to be, so that regardless of our circumstances with our family of origin we can build the sort of family we have always wanted and needed (Coleman, 1992; Sanders, 1996).

When I work with Jane I always have to keep in mind that there are many meanings of family for her. One meaning is her family of origin: her parents, siblings, and extended family. This is a large family with many aunts, uncles, and cousins spread across the Prairie Provinces in Canada. Family celebrations such as reunions, marriages, and deaths are well-attended and a source of enjoyment and encouragement for Jane.

For her, family is also her son and the young men with whom she partners. She is desperately seeking a stable partner for herself. None of these relationships yet work, because she tends to push away any partner who gets too close. Sometimes this happens because they really are not good choices. She has hooked up with some men who are violent or exploitive. One of them went to jail for several years due to a conviction on assault and drug charges. In a couple of cases she has made a good choice but struggles with the intimacy and commitment such a relationship would mean. John is a good example.

He actually dated Jane and they were not intimate for several months. He introduced her to his family and friendship circle, but Jane could not handle the normalcy of this relationship. She kept waiting for something to go wrong and in the end did push him away. I have spent a lot of time with her talking about her relationships, supporting her in them or supporting her to get out of them, sometimes confronting her about her choices and what they mean to her and her son. At times I have worked with her and the young man she is dating doing couples counselling. The program works with the fathers and the partners as much as possible.

Family is also her friends who serve family-like roles. Jane has a small circle of friends in the program who are her age. These young women have many of the same struggles. Much of the work with them is informal in that the positive attributes of the group are reinforced through casual conversation and humor can be used when the group of friends edges towards poor choices. In this way individual confidences are not compromised. As a group of friends, they support each other with advice, companionship, and babysitting. It serves the role of an extended family without really being one.

Jane also has a professional family. There have been people in her life from an early age with whom she has made a significant emotional connection, and Jane continues to visit with them and keep them up to date on her progress in life. These people mentor Jane and have earned her trust. They may never know how important they are to this young person but they are nevertheless important. For Jane this included a number of workers in the program as well as a public health nurse.

PRACTICES OF CHILD AND YOUTH CARE WORK WITH FAMILIES

Jane's story and, ultimately, that of her son can be seen as chapters of a book where multiple authors describe what happened but no one author has integrated the story. It is sometimes the case that the role of the child and youth care worker is to be that author and provide the linkages, continuity, and longevity in therapeutic relationships (Garfat, 1998). We can draw a number of conclusions from these stories about Jane in terms of what forms the core of child and youth care family work. We do not mean to imply that each of the following points will be evident in every interaction one has with clients, but over a period of time you would be likely to see evidence of them.

Physically Go to the Client Rather than Having Them Come to You

Traditional family work takes place in the counsellor's office, which is convenient for them but rarely so for the client (Ballantyne, MacDonald, & Raymond, 1998). For Jane, most of the interventions took place in her parent's home, on the phone, or at the school she attended. We believe that going to the client's world is critical. We need to interact with them where they live so as to see the real persons. In the safety of our office we are likely to see only who they want us to see. If life happens in the real world then that is where change should also happen. That is not to say that one should never see clients in your office. Sometimes that is the safest place. However, we believe that in order to truly understand the reality of the client one has to go where they live. For example, to appreciate the need for Jane to establish her own household there was a need to visit her parents' house. Such visits increase the likelihood that we understand the needs of the client.

Change Occurs in Manageable Chunks

Many of us wish for dramatic change in clients. Those are the "aha" moments you see in the movies when the therapist sets the stage through his or her brilliance for the client to have a monumental insight that changes his or her life. The client leaves the office and lives happily ever after. In real life this does not often happen. We work with people who have chaos, trauma, and pain in their lives. Much of this has gone on for a long time, and it is not realistic that one intervention will change that reality. That is not to say that you have to work for years with the family to create change. Brief interventions do work, although what is most likely needed is a series of brief interventions that are tied together in a long-term plan (Garfat, 1998).

Whether it is a series of short-term interventions or a longer-term one, the key is to break the change process into smaller, manageable components within which the client has a greater chance of achieving success. In this way the small successes build up over time into a larger change.

When one feels trapped in a seemingly unchangeable life circumstance, it is difficult to imagine an alternative view and, therefore, difficult to see a reason to try. In Jane's case, at one time everyone, including herself, focused on what was not working in her life. In order for her to gain control of her life she needed to experience some success. For her it began with success in school and in her growing sense of competency as a parent, even if in very small steps.

Interventions Are Based upon the Reality of the Client

There has to be a match between the interventions we use and the needs of the client (Charles, 1996; De Jong & Berg, 2002). There is a tendency amongst some practitioners to expect the clients to fit into the intervention rather than have a range of interventions that change based upon the needs of the client. Clients who do not fit the mold are labelled as resistant or discharged from our programs. As is shown by Jane, a rigid adherence to a particular orientation would not have served her well. In fact, without a high level of creativity and flexibility along with an ability to admit that something is not working, Jane would have disengaged from the program right at the beginning of the attempts to work with her. We should do what works when it works but stop using it when it does not. Flexibility of practice is what best helps our clients. Rigid adherence to a particular theory or intervention does not serve our clients well. Another way to say this is that interventions follow the client rather than the clients following the intervention.

Intervention Involves Advocacy

Many of the clients with whom we work have safety and living needs that must be dealt with before any other issues in their lives can be addressed. In this sense child and youth care practice needs to go beyond just dealing with the psychological, behavioral, and emotional needs that are the focus of traditional therapy. For example, Jane needed someone who could help her negotiate living conditions with her parents. Another important area of advocacy is helping clients negotiate the institutional systems in their lives. Jane needed help to work productively and cooperatively with the child protection systems, including learning to help and stick up for herself. This requires that we help our clients appreciate the strengths that they already have and to acquire the skills they need to live healthy lives (Sheafor, Horejsi, & Horejsi, 2000). With Jane this took the form of helping her acquire parenting skills and academic skills. It also meant assisting her to learn to maneuver through the many systems she contacted.

We believe it is important in child and youth care practice to move beyond a traditional definition of family and the traditional definition of what constitutes a good family. As can be seen in Jane's experience, she had a series of "families" that at least influenced her but also in many cases supported her. Her family of origin had many problems. Her mother was frequently inaccessible because of her mental illness. Her father was often overwhelmed by the demands in his life, not the least being trying to raise a large family with limited resources. Yet with all these difficulties her family tried to support her when they could and in the manner they could. One could say that this was not much and that many of Jane's troubles stemmed from her family. That may have been the case when she was younger, but that would be a static view of the situation. Regardless of what had happened in the past, her family was trying in their own way to support her in the present. At the very least they were trying to help her make the transition from their home to one of her own.

In addition, Jane was building her own family with her son. With support from many people she has been learning to become a parent. This has not been without struggles, but the important element has been her desire to give her son the sense of family that she herself did not believe she experienced as a child. At times she had young men moving in and out of her life and, in some ways, they were part of her new family. Each of us, as we grow into adults, make this transition from family of origin to what will constitute our family. This may or may not include our family of origin but will almost always include people such as friends who would not fit into a traditional definition of family. This family of choice is more fluid than a family of origin in that people move in and out of it more rapidly than in a family of origin. For Jane at this point in time this family includes some of the other young women and their children who are in the program. We believe that child and youth care family work needs to include members of the family of choice in order to be impactful (Sanders, 1996).

We also need to recognize that there is a "family of practitioners" that develops around clients on at least a temporary basis. This family is made up of all the team members and helping partners who are either directly or indirectly interacting with the client. This is clearly beneficial to the client as it provides a richer pool of expertise for the client to access at any given time. It is also beneficial for the practitioner because it supports him or her in supporting clients who at times can be demanding and draining. The more support the practitioner receives the more he or she can support the client.

Engagement Can Take a Long Time So You Have to Work at It

Patience is a major component of child and youth care family practice and in individual and group work (Ballantyne, MacDonald, & Raymond, 1998). Many of our clients are not voluntary. Many clients have no reason to trust us. They have not only been hurt as children by the adults around them, but many have also been ill-served by well-meaning professionals who have come into their lives, made glorious promises, and then disappeared when the clients did not live up to their expectations or when they appeared to be resistant to change. We need to be aware of this when we work with families.

Trust only comes through deed and action rather than through words. It does not matter who we believe ourselves to be as professionals. We have to show ourselves to our clients, and for people who have experienced the harshness of the world, trust is built is slowly over time through relationship. Every interaction is a test of the worker's integrity. Fail a test through a misstep or a broken promise or commitment and you go back to step one. Pass the test and there is likely to be another to follow shortly afterwards. Engagement can take a long time and in order for it to happen we have to work at the relationship.

Interventions Are Respectful of the Client

It is our experience that clients too often experience helping as a manipulative process within which some person who they do not believe really knows them decides that they have to work on this problem or that problem. At other times clients are given the often none too subtle message that they are bad people, bad parents, bad children or just bad. We are not suggesting that many of our clients have not made bad decisions in their lives or that they do not have long-term difficulties. However, they do not usually need to hear this from us. They already know that things are not going well and indeed their opinion of themselves is lower than the opinion anyone else can have of them. Rather than seeing helping as a positive experience, many clients view it as just one more invalidation. As can be expected, this does not lead to the kind of change that we hope for with our clients. Interventions need to be respectful of the client (De Jong & Berg, 2002; Kottler, 1991).

Jane had this experience with many helpers over the years. Her response to helpers was to either ignore them, withdraw from them, or to manipulate them. What she had not experienced was being in a relationship with helpers who acknowledged her as a person and who had some sense of the skills she had already developed in her life. Respect then involves trying to understand the person's life from their perspective rather than from the viewpoint of a rigid sense of right or wrong. As can be seen with Jane, this respect makes it possible to also have clear boundaries. Included as part of having clear boundaries also means confronting Jane when she does not follow through with her commitments and responsibilities or when she engages in self-destructive behaviors. Respect in child and youth care family practice is maintaining a balance between unconditional support and dignified confrontation.

Change Occurs Through the Relationship Rather than Through Any Specific Intervention

As we look for the one answer to the problems of all our clients we forget that no one yet has come up with a theory or model of practice that fits the reality of all of the people we encounter in our practice. Despite what we are taught in school, there is not a theory or a model or a paradigm that explains everything and, if we were being honest with ourselves, many of the ones by which we operate do not do a very good job of explaining anything. We need to keep in mind that theories–just like programs–are for our use rather than that of the clients. They provide us with a framework for our interventions but do little for the client in that sense. The relationship we develop with our clients is what creates change, not some grand intervention of the day that we all rush off to learn so that we can show the world how brilliant we are. Change comes from relationships and relationships are about human interaction (Coady, 1993; Garfat, 1998; Fewster, 1990a, 1990b; Milner, 2002).

There Is an Ebb and Flow to the Relationship Based on the Needs of the Client

It is important to be goal-focused in our interactions with clients. Indeed, if we are not working with them toward a mutually agreed upon goal, then there is little purpose in the relationship. It is not part of our professional responsibilities to engage with our clients without having a stated purpose to the relationship. They can develop less intrusive relationships with other people for the kind of non-professional supports they need in their lives. However, while keeping this in mind, it is important to realize that it is impossible and probably not healthy to try to keep a high level of intensity going in the professional relationship. Too much intensity for too long a time period can serve to overwhelm the client rather than bring him or her closer. It therefore becomes critical to understand and accept the importance of recognizing the ebb and flow or rhythmicity of relationships in order in part to understand the push and pull involved in working with people (Maier, 1992).

This natural ebb and flow is particularly important to be aware of when working with someone with Jane's background. People who have been traumatized and marginalized foremost need to develop a sense of mastery over their lives (Charles, 1996). Part of this mastery is developed through having a degree of control over the relationships in their lives in a way they have not likely experienced in the past. When the natural ebb and flow of relationships is coupled with this need for mastery the result is a movement in and out of the professional relationship based upon what is best for the client rather than the artificial requirements based upon program demands or some mistaken theory about the amount of time a practitioner and a client should spend together in a given week or month. In this case Jane needed to move in and out of the relationship based upon what she could handle at any given time and her needs.

There Is an Acknowledgement of Past Issues but Intervention Is Based upon the Present Needs of the Client

The past does have an impact upon who we are today but it is really not the reality of the past that is important but rather how we give meaning to it that is critical. In some circles it is believed that the intervention of choice with people who have been abused is to spend a great deal of time getting them to talk in detail about their traumatic experiences. This involves what some would consider a process of traumatizing the person all over again as they remember all that has happened to them (Charles, 1996). Other than maintaining them in a position of victimization, and keeping them in counselling relationship for extended periods of time, we can see no purpose in this rehashing of their pain.

The same applies to families. There is always an issue that can be rehashed over and over, resulting in the family never moving forward. We believe that in child and youth care practice interventions need to focus upon what people need to live their lives today and into tomorrow. Jane had a history with a long list of horror stories. Rehashing these would have not served to help her in her academic quests or make her an effective parent. What Jane needed was help in learning how to get the most out of the present for herself and her son. This is not to say that you want to ignore the past. Rather, it is to say that what is important about the past is only how it impacts how you function in the present.

Change Occurs in the Developmental Context of the Client's Life

Without suggesting a particular developmental theory, we believe that a child and youth care approach also must take into account the developmental stage of the family and of the individuals in the family. This notion of "applied developmental intervention" is keyed upon the understanding that people, families, and systems change over time and, as they do, so do their needs. Development in this sense is never static. However, a person or family may have age-appropriate development in one area while remaining developmentally delayed in another. One can have great analytical skills but not be able to interact in a mature manner with their family members. Developmental maturity in any one area can also move forward or retreat depending upon the external and internal pressures being experienced by the family, person, or system. Enough pressure can cause a regression in skills or views of the world resulting in a movement back to an earlier way of coping. This is the "two steps forward, one step back" dynamic that we so often see with our clients in times of stress. It is also important to place this developmental perspective into an ecological context in order to truly begin to understand why people do what they do when they do it (Coleman, 1992; Garbarino & Eckenrode, 1997; Goldner, 1985). Cultural, societal, and family expectations and belief systems can impact upon how one develops and matures. In Jane's case one of her struggles was to overcome the underlying messages in her family that women have to be sick to get attention or their needs met. This was not necessarily how her mother viewed the world, but it does appear to be the message that Jane picked up from her family. It will take a great effort on her part to move from this passive way of interacting with the world into a manner of interacting that is more adult and mature.

CONCLUSION

Child and youth care is in the process of developing a unique way of working with families that goes beyond traditional forms of intervention. It is unique in that it is not limited to one theoretical viewpoint or a single way of intervening. Rather, family work in child and youth care practice builds upon our rich history of working with our clients towards a common goal through multiple pathways. In this sense child and work care family practice involves utilizing a range of flexible interactions that are based upon the needs of our clients rather than a set program or way of doing things. Child and youth care practice is about respecting and encouraging our clients to gain mastery over their lives. It is about being supportive in a planned way. It involves being with our clients in their lives at the times they need us. Child and youth care practice is about helping our clients see the greater picture of their lives and learning to fully participate in it. Family work in child and youth care practice is a way of being with clients where they are and when they are so that we work in their reality. It is these principles that form the foundation of our work.

REFERENCES

Austin, D., & Halpin, W. (1989). The caring response. *Journal of Child and Youth Care,* *4*(3), 1-7.

Ballantyne, M., MacDonald, G., & Raymond, L. (1998). Fundamental processes for interventions: Working with high-risk adolescents and their families. *Journal of Child and Youth Care, 12*(3), 69-81.

Charles, G. (1996). *Experiences of extreme abuse.* Unpublished doctoral dissertation, University of Victoria, Victoria, British Columbia, Canada.

Coady, N. F. (1993, May). The worker-client relationship revisited. *Families in Society: The Journal of Contemporary Human Services,* 291-298.

Coleman, H. (1992). "Good families don't . . ." and other family myths. *Journal of Child and Youth Care, 7*(2), 59-67.

De Jong, P., & Berg, I. K. (2002). *Interviewing for solutions (2nd ed.).* Pacific Grove CA: Brooks/Cole.

Dolan, Y. M. (1991). *Resolving sexual abuse: Solution-focused therapy and Ericksonian hypnosis for adult survivors.* New York: W. W. Norton and Company.

Fewster, G. (1990a). *Being in care: A journey into self.* New York: The Haworth Press, Inc.

Fewster, G. (1990b). Growing together: The personal relationship in child and youth care. In C. Denholm, R. Ferguson, & A. Pence (Eds.), *Professional child and youth care practice: Part 1* (pp. 25-40). New York: The Haworth Press, Inc.

Fox, L. E. (1994). The catastrophe of compliance. *Journal of Child and Youth Care, 9*(1), 13-21.

Garbarino, J., & Eckenrode, J. (1997). The meaning of maltreatment. In J. Garbarino & J. Eckenrode (Eds.), *Understanding abusive families* (pp. 3-25). San Francisco: Jossey-Bass.

Garfat, T. (1998). The effective child and youth care intervention: A phenomenological inquiry. *Journal of Child and Youth Care, 12*(1-2), 5-178.

Goldner, V. (1985). Feminism and family therapy. *Family Process, 24*(1), 31-47.

Kottler, J. A. (1991). *The compleat therapist.* San Francisco: Jossey-Bass.

Krueger, M. A. (1991). Coming from your center, being there, meeting them where they're at, interacting together, counseling on the go, creating circles of caring, discovering and using self, and caring for one another: Central themes in professional child and youth care. *Journal of Child and Youth Care, 5*(1), 77-87.

Maier, H. W. (1992). Rhythmicity: A powerful force for experiencing unity and personal connections. *Journal of Child and Youth Care, 5*(1), 7-13.

Milner, R. (2002). Promoting health or curing illness: A child and youth care approach to mental health. *Journal of Child and Youth Care, 15*(1), 43-51.

Pearce, J. W., & Pezzot-Pearce, T. D. (1997). *Psychotherapy of abused and neglected children.* New York: The Guilford Press.

Pennell J., & Burford, G. (1994). Widening the circle: Family group decision making. *Journal of Child and Youth Care, 9*(1), 1-11.

Philion, C. A. (2002). A legacy for the millennium: Two hundred years of systemic abuse of children in substitute care. *Journal of Child and Youth Care, 15*(1), 33-41.

Ross, A., & Hoeltke, G. (1987). An interview model for selecting residential child care workers. *Child Welfare, 66*(2), 175-183.

Sanders, G. L. (1996). Recovering from paraphilia: An adolescent's journey from despair to hope. *Journal of Child and Youth Care, 11*(1), 43-54.

Sheafor, B. W., Horejsi, C. R., & Horejsi, G. A. (2000). *Techniques and guidelines for social work practice (5th ed.).* Boston: Allyn and Bacon.

Walsh, F. (2002, April). A family resilience framework: Innovative practice applications. *Family Relations: Interdisciplinary Journal of Applied Family Studies, 51*(2), 130-137.

Knowing:
The Critical Error
of Ethics in Family Work

Frances Ricks
Gerrard Bellefeuille

SUMMARY. When working with families, family workers are expected to know what to do in order to practice ethically. The key for family workers staying open to inquiry and ethical endeavor is for family workers to understand *how they know what they know*. By understanding how they know what they know they can avoid making premature assumptions of what they do not know. Promoting a collective awareness of self and others within family can be used to inform the family of how they operate and can be used to formulate and create an evolving ethic that can be lived by the family. *[Article copies available for a fee from The Haworth Document Delivery Service: 1-800-HAWORTH. E-mail address: <docdelivery@haworthpress.com> Website: <http://www.HaworthPress.com> © 2003 by The Haworth Press, Inc. All rights reserved.]*

KEYWORDS. Youthwork with families, youth care work, social work with families, family-centered residential care, child and youth care, family services, family support, parent education, residential care work and families

Frances Ricks is affiliated with the University of Victoria. Gerrard Bellefeuille is affiliated with the University of Northern British Columbia.

[Haworth co-indexing entry note]: "Knowing: The Critical Error of Ethics in Family Work." Ricks, Frances, and Gerrard Bellefeuille. Co-published simultaneously in *Child & Youth Services* (The Haworth Press, Inc.) Vol. 25, No. 1/2, 2003, pp. 117-130; and: *A Child and Youth Care Approach to Working with Families* (ed: Thom Garfat) The Haworth Press, Inc., 2003, pp. 117-130. Single or multiple copies of this article are available for a fee from The Haworth Document Delivery Service [1-800-HAWORTH, 9:00 a.m. - 5:00 p.m. (EST). E-mail address: docdelivery@haworthpress.com].

Family workers perceive, interpret, and deal with life experiences within family practice that is shaped by their internal maps of reality or what they think is true about reality.

The internal map is based on paradigms or mental models (Senge, 1995) that shape thoughts, feelings, and actions. Kuhn (1962) notes that every time something is beyond the boundaries of personal paradigms or maps, it is not possible to see the opportunities that lie beyond. This point is demonstrated in the following folklore:

> A man was speeding down a dusty and twisty country road in his fancy red sports car. It was a sunny and bright day. He had the top down on his car and was singing out loud while feeling on top of the world. As he approached a bend in the road, out of nowhere came another car driven by a woman weaving from one lane to the other. He managed to avoid smashing into her and to his surprise, as she passed, she yelled at him, "pig." He was startled and yelled back at her "stupid woman!" as she sped down the road and out of sight. He was enraged and thought, "How dare she! She called me a pig! She was the one driving all over the road!" He collected himself, breathed deeply, straightened his hat, and sped off at full speed down the road. Around the corner he smashed right into the pig.

In this story the man thought he knew that the woman was calling him a pig; therefore, it was outside his knowing to consider that she might be alerting him to the danger of running into a pig around the corner.

It is our premise that ethical practice is construed and driven by the importance placed on having requisite knowledge within a particular practice culture because such knowledge is supposed to inform what ethical practice is and how to conduct it. We argue that knowing sometimes prevents family workers from being open to exploring the complexity of ethics within family work; hence knowing is a critical barrier to co-creating ethics and living them within family work. Further we argue, ethical practice that relies totally on professional codes of ethics and standards of practice have been based on the "knowing" paradigm and can be impediments to ethical and moral reasoning within the practice context. Such codes can lull practitioners to sleep in matters that require critical reflection and discretionary judgment with regard to families and communities. Finn (1994) explains it this way: "Ethics which rely on the (political) categories of established thought and/or seeks to solidify or cement them . . . into institutionalized rights and freedoms, rules and regulations, and principles of practice . . . is not so much an ethic as an abdication of ethics for politics under another description" (p. 101).

Doing away with knowledge, rules and codes is not a solution. Rather, we challenge the reader to be alert to the limitations of rule-based formulations in family work as an attempt to deal with the unknown. We encourage family workers to be open to inquiry and on-going learning as a means to creating an ethical inquiry that prompts discovery and learning within the family. We offer some ideas and frameworks that link the ethical endeavors of family workers and family members to family or community relationships. These ideas and frameworks offer ways to explore different perspectives on what family workers might want to know, how to know it, and how to inquire collectively into the unique family or community issues that require unique and ever-changing perspectives.

ETHICAL ENDEAVOR AS ETHICAL PRACTICE

The practice of ethics in the context of working with families in community is not easily defined or understood. Ethics refers to a set of moral principles to live by, and professional ethics are those principles for professional conduct that are used to guide practitioners in making ethical choices. Gray (1993) posits that practitioners see ethical choices as being situations perceived as being out of control. Alternatively, ethical issues have been simply represented as concerns with how people are behaving, such as the behavior of particular family or community members, usually contrary to the cultural norm.

Blum (1994) has summarized key differences in framing ethical concerns and how to handle them, drawing on the competing views of leading theorists such as Kohlberg and Gilligan. He notes:

1. the impartial rationalist versus the care-responsibility approach,
2. not needing to know the other versus needing to understand the significance of all persons as the focus of ethical and moral concern,
3. appreciating the complexity of ethical concerns which are informed by love, care, empathy, compassion, and sensitivity versus informed by formal rationality,
4. the use of non-subjective standards to appraise a particular situation versus using such standards to generate rules of behavior to control practice, and
5. the need or not for connections and direct responses between persons involved in the situation in order to express and sustain the connections of all parties to each other.

These comparisons make explicit that some formulations of ethics in practice focus on achieving a rational understanding of how to make correct choices using a set of universal standards and to correct them when "poor choices" have been made. Achieving a rational understanding of what to do usually involves some form of codes of ethics or standards of practice. Family workers are prompted to ask, "What should we do in this case? How is this case similar or dissimilar to other cases? What are the values that we need to maintain consistency across cases? Have professional standards of practice been violated and should someone be punished?"

More recent formulations suggest that ethical concerns are only in relation to the self and cannot be separated from the self and the context of the situation (Blum, 1994; Flanagan & Jackson, 1987; Ricks & Charlesworth, 2002; Sharmer, 2000). Blum (1994) argues that the ethical or moral[1] particularly involves "getting oneself to attend to the reality of individual other persons . . . while not allowing one's own needs, bias, fantasies (conscious and unconscious), and desires regarding the other persons to get in the way of appreciating his or her own particular needs and situation" (p. 12). With this focus on attending to the other, ethical endeavor requires making a deliberate attempt to determine *good human conduct* toward the other, or put another way, ethical and moral comportment evolves and unfolds within the context of relationship and is created within relationship.

From this point of view personal relationships provide the principal setting in which ethical or moral endeavor takes place and involve a concerned responsiveness to others in the situation. Family workers are engaged in concerned and deliberate responsiveness to people in particular situations in every situation in family and community practice. Family workers can only be more deliberate when they are aware of how they see the world–aware of their paradigms–how they know what they know, as well as understanding the capacity and manifestations of care such as compassion, concern, love, friendship and kindness in order to understand the other's situation (Murdoch, 1983). Critical to engaging in this kind of care is the need to be self-aware while co-creating a context of care (Garfat & Ricks, 1995) within family practice.

Personal relationships as the ethical context of practice has been previously identified within the field of child and youth care by students who studied ethical dilemmas within practicum settings (Ricks, 1997). These students concluded from an analysis of their dilemmas that ethical practice was less about the lofty determination of right from wrong and more about the common experience of endeavoring to be personal while engaging in a process of ethical reasoning, moral thinking, and personal determination of what matters. Most importantly, they concluded that ethical endeavor requires being able to act on that determination. The following examples illustrate how these students had the common experience of not being able to act on doing the right thing for reasons of personal fear. These examples clearly exemplify how the contextual factors influence how child and youth practitioners respond, even when knowing "the right thing to do."

Helen was a student in a practicum setting that involved the care of young children. After observing a drunken father pick up his daughter a number of times she reported this to the owner/director. The director said she would take care of it. The situation worsened and the student said nothing more as she feared for her practicum and potential job opportunity.

A female employee in a center for emotionally disturbed children was putting up with sexual overtures from an immediate supervisor. She was a single mother who needed the employment. The supervisor suggested one day that he could "help" her get a supervisory position, and this was the last straw. She went to the director of the agency who refused to believe that his supervisor would be inappropriate and dismissed her allegations. Further he suggested that she needed a change in attitude. She let it drop and began looking for a new position.

A group of workers in a social services agency were sitting around at lunch engaged in "serious gossip" about other workers not present. The nature of the discussion took the form of unsubstantiated accusations of unprofessional and unethical behavior. It was agreed that such behavior should not be tolerated. One member of the group said that these accusations were not substantiated and that the group was perpetrating unprofessional and unethical behavior by participating in this discussion. This was followed by silence and soon the group broke up. The outspoken worker stopped going to the lunchroom.

Being able to take a personal stance and act on that stance in ethical practice raises questions as to the relevance of rules that are embedded in codes of ethics or standards of practice. We argued earlier that codified rules of what to do in particular cases, and cases of like kind, gets us *off the hook* of moral endeavor (Finn, 1994). Adherence to codified rules does not necessarily require self-awareness or accountability for taking a moral stance. It simply requires learning the rules and following them, whereupon we may fall prey to being lulled to sleep as we methodically attempt to capture similarities across cases and avoid the unique complexities of the situation at hand. In the earlier stories it is apparent that all three people could have spoken out or done something, and they did not.

The family worker's regard for codes and standards will play a significant role in how the family worker guides the family sessions and will likely influence choices made by the family members as they work together. However, the codes and standards are only part of the contextual mix used by the family worker and are differentially applied in practice. The challenge for the family worker is to be mindful of all the factors, including codes and standards, while engaging family members in a process of creating family relationships that allows for and reflects the sharing of values for participation and change. For example, consider other factors as current institutional practice, legal obligations, customary social practices, unpredictable contextual influences, and unknown offshoots or consequences (DeMarco, 1997). In consideration of these many factors, family workers use the codes and standards for what they are, guidelines or standards held as important by the professional organization that produced them. Such codes and standards must be considered as part of the complex context of moral endeavor that is influenced by the many factors that need to be taken into account. It is within the relationship with the family that the family worker promotes the sharing, understanding, and living of values that results in the family being able to create new ways for being together.

FAMILIES IN COMMUNITY

Shifting ethical and moral endeavor as a way *to be in practice* with family or community members alters the purpose of family work. Rather than focusing on *changing the family's behavior*, the family worker assists the family in co-creating an ethos or attitude of how to be within the family culture. This involves a paradigm shift in thinking from individual moral endeavor to community moral endeavor as well as a shift in focus from *what the family does* to *how the family thinks* of itself as a community of relationships.

Those who work with families in communities will readily identify the complexities involved when moving from *me to we*. In addition there is the complexity of co-creating the culture in which the family can agree to live differently together. This requires an understanding of world views, values, and what works and what does not for all persons engaged in the process whether they are directly or indirectly involved, specifically, other practitioners involved in the case. It also requires a great deal of awareness and understanding of how the family worker sees him or herself in relation to others, and how they are in their relationships with family members and others.

By family or community we are referring to a collection of relationships and their collective values that provide the context in which we live our lives, hopefully lives of health and wellbeing (Ricks, Charlesworth, Bellefeuille, & Field, 1999). It is within family and community relationships that we recognize each other and this recognition is significant to the personal formation, development, and sustainability of the ethical and moral selves. The recognition and identification within community and our relationship to community has the effect of shaping our sense of what we are "morally pulled to do and . . . what is and is not an undue burden or too much to demand" (Blum, 1994, p. 145). MacIntyre (1984) attributes links between ethical endeavor and community endeavor to the learning that occurs within social life, including family life, and suggests that moral identity and agency is a function of and sustained by the communities of which we are members. Using a business metaphor, John Morse (1999) says,

> Business cannot be thought of as an entity whose practices, goals, and purposes are separate and different from the goals, purposes and practices of the communities within which they find themselves. Rather, a business should be conceived as a moral entity that is necessarily situated within a community and contributes to the good of the whole community. It follows that as a moral member of the community, a business must realize that it has a profound influence on the formation of the members of the community through the cultivation of desires and by encouraging and discouraging various kinds of moral behaviors. (p. 48)

In other words, the ethos of the family or community or the characteristic attitudes or paradigms of the family influence our individual and collective participation in ethical endeavors to create change.

In the three situations described earlier, all three students experienced the undue burden of doing the best thing when confronted by what they considered to be too much to demand from them. These students were burdened by needing to do the right thing and were not able to do so. They were ill prepared to tackle these issues within the context of being in relationships and were unable to approach the issues with understanding of the other. They tried to sustain an impartial and rational stance and were ill unprepared to deal with their emotional reality within the on-going relationships.

THE RELEVANCE OF HOW WE KNOW WHAT WE KNOW

Given this link between individual and community ethical endeavor it is imperative that when working with families and communities, family workers are mindful of the messages they send to family and community members. By being mindful, they can avoid confusing their needs and situations with those of the other members of community. Being mindful enables workers to respect differences and helps to resolve value conflicts that are inevitable within families and communities. However, *knowing* can get us into trouble.

To *know* as family workers is to be aware and to be informed. Usually family workers take what they know as representing what is true and, in light of that truth, generate solutions to problems or reactions to previous actions. To understand one's stance on knowing and not knowing requires reflection on one's theory of knowledge, especially with regards to the methods one uses to know and to validate information. For example, family workers can know from research that has been reported in scholarly journals, through mass media, from what others tell them, from direct experiences, and from cultural traditions and rituals. Information received from any source is validated or invalidated based on personal beliefs and values of knowledge development and what is held as true. It is important to be aware and understand that family workers take in certain evidence and dismiss other evidence; they use "certain" evidence to ratify, accept, or confirm what they think they know. How they obtain this information and use it to inform practice represents what they will seek to know in practice.

To make this more concrete in practice, consider the following questions.

- What is taken as evidence for family or community membership?
- What is taken as evidence of family or community issues?
- Who gets to participate in the formulation of issues and how they get resolved?
- What sources of information inform? What sources of information are ignored or tend to be disregarded?
- What family or community members are taken more seriously and tend to be believed over others?
- Under what conditions would participation of family members or community members not be sanctioned or approved?
- How long does it take to engage with family and community?
- What are indicators of engagement, trust, cooperation and collaboration?

Answers to these kinds of questions give meaning to fundamental beliefs and values about working with families and communities. Further, they point to the evidence for what is believed to be true and provide the blueprint or map used to seek certain information or evidence. The key point is that truth and knowledge, and how it is known, informs intentional action in practice. When family workers are unaware of their truth and how they come to it, they act mindlessly and without intention.

FROM ME TO WE: PARTICIPATORY INQUIRY

Knowing becomes more complex within the context of family work because knowing involves a collective learning and understanding. In family work it is important for each knower to have an awareness of their knowing and how that influences their decisions; it is also important to be aware of others' knowing. Therefore, a key aspect of family work is to make transparent to family members how they relate and participate in family knowing. This is apparent by getting family members to pay attention to how family members organize themselves in carrying out family tasks or by observing family patterns of behavior. By recognizing how family members relate to one another within these persistent patterns, they reveal their family beliefs and values that are held individually and collectively. Very often such patterns are not explicit or transparent to family members and subsequently are not understood.

Figure 1 is a framework that might be useful in helping families identify and understand the foundation for doing what they do while teaching them how to engage with each other in mutual and collective inquiry and learning.

In Figure 1, the two inner circles represent the individual's history and knowing. As the individual participates in a participatory inquiry process, there is an interaction with all other members' histories and ways of knowing. It is at this place where the individual's experience and way of knowing intersects with other histories and ways of knowing. For example, if a person has a strong belief that only like kind (e.g., the same gender) can appreciate their issue, then not everyone can know what they know. That would have the effect of excluding others who are not of like kind from participatory learning and understanding. Another example might be when participants have different views about what constitutes learning; then there would likely be a narrowing of options in terms of what to take as evidence for collective knowing. The more participants engaged in the inquiry of their different histories and experiences, the more complex and involving it becomes. There are revelations on the part of one or some about the others, specifically, "Oh, I did not know you felt that way." "Wow, what a different perspective; I would never have seen it that way." Such revelations can lead to more inquiry: "Explain what makes you feel that way." "What led you to come to that perspective, or what makes you think that?" The journey guided by the family worker assists the family in making the implicit explicit, so that changes can be negotiated. Family members cannot change what they do not know or understand. Perhaps more important, the family and family members live a personal and collective inquiry into each others beliefs and values that in turn models or lives an ethic of caring for and learning about each other. Though this participatory inquiry and learning, family members then co-create their ethos for participation and decision-making. This is apparent in Table 1.

Table 1[2] shows that within family there can be many beliefs and values about participation and decision making. If there is to be full participation and collective ethical endeavor of all family members, family members need to tell and negotiate values to be used for future participation. Examples in Table 1 make explicit that in this particular family the collective values represent their commitment to building a context of care, being open to collective learning, and being open to collective change. Fundamental beliefs for promoting such inquiry and collaborative introspection and learning are: Everyone and every family have the capacity to participate and learn together to make collective decisions, and that change creates new opportunities for learning and change. A mutual and collective understanding of beliefs and principles for action

FIGURE 1. Moving from "Me" to "We" in the Participatory Inquiry Process

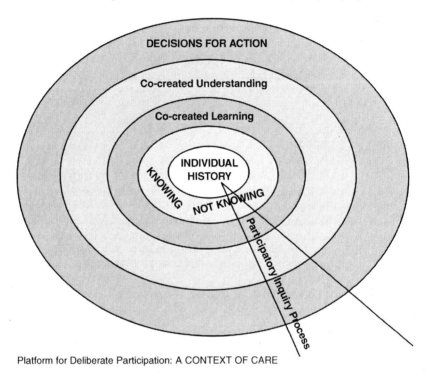

Platform for Deliberate Participation: A CONTEXT OF CARE

comes out of a collective commitment to inquiry and learning. This creates possibility and capacity for taking collective action.

What is required from family workers who are committed to promoting collective inquiry and action in family work? It takes in-depth learning of what is true and how each person determines what is true. Only by attending to the reality of each other can the family collectively come to know and be informed by the collective knowing and, in turn, be able to take collective action. When there is mutual understanding of each other's reality, the likelihood of disagreement is reduced; the understanding is simply how it is for each person. Therefore, there can now be a collective ethical endeavor since ethical endeavors are simply decisions that reflect certain value stances. By telling and discussing the values presented in Table 1, this particular family created an opportunity to discover their own principles for ethical practice and co-created an ethos of care that opens up new possibilities for collective learning and change.

TABLE 1. From Values to Principles for Community Action

Values	Principles
Love	Build a context of care
Care	
Wonder	Operate collectively by being caring/living care
Curiosity	
Deliberate expression of concern	
Participatory commitment	
Humility	Be open to collective learning (willingness)
Learning	
Tolerance	
Understanding	
Collective inquiry	Be open to collective change
Multiple perspectives/differences	
Awareness of possibilities	
Perplexity	
Purposeful	Everyone and every family has the capacity for inquiry and learning
Represents a value-based position	
Represents a commitment to inquiry and action	
Ambiguity	Change creates new opportunities for learning and change
Change	
Promise/hope/optimism	
New opportunities	
Accomplishment/satisfaction	

LIVING COLLECTIVE ETHICAL ENDEAVOR

As family workers, what can be done to promote collective ethical endeavor in families? A key element in collective ethical endeavor is conscious participation on the part of family workers in promoting collective inquiry and understanding. We propose three suggestions for conscious participation of family workers:

- Stay open to inquiry,
- Subject your beliefs of learning and knowing to critical analysis, and
- Do not succumb to or be overcome by existing conditions.

Staying open to inquiry requires maintaining the possibility of wonderment and surprise. In other words, to allow the self to be surprised, to notice the unexpected or the astonishing. Staying open to inquiry depends on suspending what is known, to suspend knowledge of previous stories in order to listen and see with *fresh eyes*. Langer (1997) argues that being open to learning requires a mindful state and that being mindful is being alert in the following ways:

a. be open to novelty,
b. be alert to distinction,
c. be sensitive to different contexts,
d. be aware of multiple perspectives, and
e. stay in the present.

In essence, come from a place of inquiry and do not make assumptions of what may be true. Not making assumptions is less difficult in the early stages of family work. As time goes on and the therapeutic relational patterns become more established, the family worker needs to be vigilant about what might be in order to stay open to new possibilities.

Subjecting beliefs of learning and knowing to critical analysis requires being able to reflect on beliefs and values in the moment. Rather than taking an early stance on what is true about the family, propose formulations, speak about the underlying assumptions embedded within them, and ask whether these are relevant to others in the family. By being aware or mindful of what they think, family workers can verify the relevance and usefulness of their beliefs within the family. By challenging family beliefs, family workers are taking responsibility for their formulations and what actions might be taken. This sharing may prompt family members to generate other possibilities. This models the inquiry process for family members and encourages them to exchange their formulations about and for each other.

Perhaps this suggestion is the most crucial: *Do not succumb to or be overcome by existing conditions*. Being overcome by conditions and succumbing to them is giving way to determinants perceived as overwhelming. It is to capitulate, to give up, to be confused, to lose the integrity of what family members consider true in the situation. It is to allow other values to take precedence in the moment even when there is compelling evidence for what to do. It may be to succumb to the virtues of training and education, rather than on the experience within the context of the family. Both individuals and collectives succumb!

In the context of family and community work, succumbing happens all the time. Succumbing may be an aspect of why, when we know the right thing to do, we do not do it. It may be because we are overwhelmed by existing conditions and fearful of now knowing what to do. For example,

James thinks that a child in this family is at risk and knows that the prevailing policy is to not take kids into care. He decides not to report the circumstances of the child, because he does not want to deal with his supervisor, fellow workers, or central office because he is not following policy. And policy is law. It's just too overwhelming.

Donna negotiates a transfer from one supervisor to another as quietly as possible, because she does not want to deal with the unions, the administration, or her family who are urging her to not make a fuss–just make it work. She decides to avoid the investigation and to get on with her life. It is too much hassle and as she is up against a system in which she will likely not be heard. So, she is silenced. It's just too overwhelming.

Families in the community put up with an impure water situation because the public officials are reassuring and report that everything is fine. This is a community where political appointees receive certain benefits that other community members do not receive. Subsequent complaints are viewed as *sour grapes*. It's just too overwhelming.

In these situations people succumbed to the pressure and were overwhelmed by what it takes to challenge the status quo. Paradoxically, they do not know what they know, or they are not prepared to act on what they know, or both.

CONCLUSION

We are proposing that ethical endeavors in family practice are complex because they require an awareness, appreciation and understanding of the larger contexts. All issues, and the decisions to resolve them within family practice, are ethical endeavors because they involve personal reflections and analysis of knowing and learning, beliefs and values on all that matters to a particular family and on what is considered virtuous or good with regard to participation and co-creating change as a family. Ethical endeavors require us to be engaged in a process of understanding the other's reality by showing care, compassion, kindness, and love while co-creating a context of care.

Moving from individual ethical endeavor to family or community ethical endeavor requires critical reflection, self-awareness, and a commitment to three key processes for participatory inquiry: stay open to inquiry, subject your beliefs of learning and knowing to critical analysis, and do not succumb to or be overcome by existing conditions. The paradoxical knowing of what to do comes out of not knowing while being willing to inquire while co-creating a process of inquiry and learning.

NOTES

1. Moral philosophy is the branch of philosophy having to do with ethics, therefore, we use the terms ethical and moral interchangeably.

2. Figure 1 and Table 1 were created for the Participatory Inquiry Project, Child Care Federation of Canada, Ottawa, 2001. This project was funded by Human Resources Canada.

REFERENCES

Banister, E. (1999). Evolving reflexivity: Negotiating meaning of women's midlife experience. *Qualitative Inquiry, 5*(1), 3-23.

Blum, L. (1994). *Moral perception and particularity.* Cambridge: Cambridge University Press.

DeMarco, J. (1997). Coherence and applied ethics. *Journal of Applied Philosophy, 14*(3), 289-300.

Finn, G. (1994). The space-between ethics and politics: Or more of the same? In L. Godway & G. Finn (Eds.), *Who is this "We"? Absence of community* (pp. 101-115). Montreal: Black Rose Books Limited.

Flanagan, O., & Jackson, L. (1987). Justice, care and gender: The Kohlberg-Gilligan debate revisited. *Ethics 97*, 622-37.

Garfat, T., & Ricks, F. (1995). Self-driven ethical decision-making: A model for child and youth care. *Child and Youth Care Forum, 24*(6), 393-404.

Gilligan, Carol (1982). *In a different voice.* Cambridge, MA: Harvard University Press.

Gray, M. (1993). *The relationship between social work, ethics and politics.* Unpublished doctoral dissertation. University of Natal, Durban.

Gray, M. (1995). The ethical implications of current theoretical developments in social work. *British Journal of Social Work, 25*(1), 55-70.

Kohlberg, L. (1981). *Essays on moral development in the philosophy of moral development.* New York: Harper & Row.

Kuhn, T. (1962). *The structure of scientific revolutions.* Chicago, IL: University of Chicago Press.

Langer, E. (1997). *The power of mindful learning.* Cambridge, MA: Perseus Books.

MacIntyre, A. (1984). Is patriotism a virtue? (The Lindley Lecture), University of Kansas.

Morse, J. (1999). The missing link between virtue theory and business ethics. *Journal of Applied Philosophy, 16*(11), 47-58.

Murdoch, I. (1970). *The sovereignty of good.* London: Routledge and Kegan Paul.

Ricks, F. (1997). Perspectives on ethics in child and youth care. *Child and Youth Care Forum, 26*(3), 187-204.

Ricks, F., & Charlesworth, J. (2002). *Emergent practice planning.* New York: Kluwer Academic/Plenum Publishers.

Ricks, F., Charlesworth, J., Bellefeuille, G., & Field, A. (1999). *All together now: Creating a social capital mosaic.* Victoria, BC: Morris Printing Company Ltd.

Scharmer, C. O. (2000). *Presencing: Learning from the future as it emerges. On the tacit dimension of leading revolutionary change.* Paper presented at the Conference on Knowledge and Innovation, Helsinki School of Economics, Finland, May 25-26, 2000.

Activity-Oriented Family-Focused Child and Youth Work in Group Care: Integrating Streams of Thought into a River of Progress

Karen VanderVen

SUMMARY. Three streams of thought are important, including a general concept of family-focused work, the centrality of relationship in development and, increasingly in child and youth care work, activity and activity programming. Activity-oriented family-focused work builds on working in the life space of the child and his family to consider what family members do together, how those activities contribute to or inhibit development and family relationships, and expanded possibilities for the worker's relationship with the members of the family. *[Article copies available for a fee from The Haworth Document Delivery Service: 1-800-HAWORTH. E-mail address: <docdelivery@haworthpress.com> Website: <http://www.HaworthPress.com> © 2003 by The Haworth Press, Inc. All rights reserved.]*

KEYWORDS. Youthwork with families, youth care work, social work with families, family-centered residential care, child and youth care, family services, family support, parent education, residential care work and families

Karen VanderVen is affiliated with the University of Pittsburgh.

[Haworth co-indexing entry note]: "Activity-Oriented Family-Focused Child and Youth Work in Group Care: Integrating Streams of Thought into a River of Progress." VanderVen, Karen. Co-published simultaneously in *Child & Youth Services* (The Haworth Press, Inc.) Vol. 25, No. 1/2, 2003, pp. 131-147; and: *A Child and Youth Care Approach to Working with Families* (ed: Thom Garfat) The Haworth Press, Inc., 2003, pp. 131-147. Single or multiple copies of this article are available for a fee from The Haworth Document Delivery Service [1-800-HAWORTH, 9:00 a.m. - 5:00 p.m. (EST). E-mail address: docdelivery@haworthpress.com].

Intramural school is over in the residential treatment center. The youth struggle back onto their living unit and flop on the couch. "It's so boring around here," sighs one bystander. Soon a few are gazing glassy-eyed at the television set. Several others begin to scuffle with each other until the staff come out of the staff room and intervene. As the melee escalates, a senior worker yells, "And for this your home visits for this weekend are cancelled!"

"He just lies around all day watching television all day," laments Mrs. Smith to the child and youth care worker making a home visit regarding Jimmy, age 11. "And when he's not doing that, he just gets into mischief. I don't know what to do with him."

"Oh, I'm just so discouraged." says Josie's mother to Josie's "key" child and youth worker on a visit to her living unit. "There's just so much I have to deal with; sometimes I wonder how I can go on." Mother's appearance and demeanor support her statements: Her hair is straggly, her complexion gray, and her clothing indifferently put together.

"Now, to improve Joey's acting out and "hyper" behavior, let's set up a reward system," states Mr. Jones, a counselor, to Joey's mother and father who are seated in his office. "First, we'll identify those behaviors that will be reinforced. For each of them you will tell Joey what he must do and what will result in non-reinforcement. Then for each we'll set up an allocation of points to be given when you observe each of these behaviors." He continues, not realizing that he lost the attention of the parents a long time ago.

The above vignettes represent situations that today's child and youth care workers could encounter when working in a family-focused group care setting. There has been some attention given to how families can be reached and involved in group care through utilization of activities. However, the potential power of such an approach that is congruent with past and current advances in conceptualizing and practicing in the field of child and youth work perhaps has not been stated. On the premise that a more articulated integration of *activity-based* approaches into contemporary child and youth care work with families will advance the scope of the field and the effectiveness of family work, this chapter will:

1. Identify three fundamental streams of thought in child and youth work that can be woven into a new conception of the role of activities in family work.
2. Describe relevant concepts from the past decade or so that can extend and enrich the conceptualization of activity-oriented, family-focused child and youth care work.
3. Describe what activity oriented family-focused work looks like.

BACKGROUND

Over the past 25 years or so, streams of theory and practice have evolved that contribute to increasing recognition of the importance of family-focused child and youth work and the role of activity in development, and there have been some efforts to utilize activities in family focused practice. Three basic streams underlie this attempt to formulate an integrated contemporary conception of family-focused child and youth care work: the general concept of family-focused work, the centrality of relationship in development and, increasingly, in child and youth care work activity and activity programming. Because these have been described extensively elsewhere, they will only be highlighted here to establish an initial framework for an extended and contemporary model for family-focused activity centered child and youth care work.

Family-Focused Child and Youth Care Work

Over the past decade, it has become increasingly recognized that to "treat" a child without including and supporting the family is much less effective without family involvement. To this end, a literature showing how the competency areas associated with the profession of child and youth work can be applied in work with families, for example, Ainsworth (1997), Anglin (1984), Garfat (2002), VanderVen (1987, 1991), and VanderVen and Stuck (1996). Among the major themes are ways that child and youth workers can work with families in their daily lives to gain the support and services that will enable them to better raise children, and how strategies that workers use to encourage positive behavior in children might also be adapted by their families.

Relationship in Human Development

In recent years, the centrality of relationship building and relationship as developmental support and intervention has been emphasized in the field of human development. Such concepts as attachment dynamics (Maier, 1987), social perspective taking (Selman, Watts, & Schultz, 1997), interpersonal communication (Goleman, 1995) and the evolution of self (Harter, 1999) have all been considered in the context of forming and maintaining beneficial relationships. Because many of the children and youth served by child and youth workers have experienced many barriers to the development of attachment, social skills, and a positive self-identity, over the past years child and youth work has increasingly identified *relationships* as an important concern. VanderVen (1999) described this approach as *relational child and youth care* using as major sources the formulations of Fewster (1990), Garfat (1998), and Krueger (1998).

Major features of relational child and youth care are:

- The relationship between the child/child and youth care worker is the central mediator in that youth's development and is forged in mutuality, rhythmicity, and caregiving interactions.
- The process and synchronicity of interaction . . . is the way in which positive development is encouraged through the relationship that evolves.
- The personhood and selfhood are admissible into the relationship.
- The interaction occurs "in the moment" which is multiply determined by the attributes of the participants and the context.

Because real relationship in the context of daily living is indeed such a fundamental force in human development, and because the structure and content of other human service professions has deemphasized both relationship quality and intervention in the life space, this is a transformational advance showing the uniqueness and significance of "care" work.

Activity and Activity Programming

As with the formation of real relationships in the daily life space of the client, the role of *activity* (e.g., play, sports, games, arts and crafts, music, service, dramatics) in development has generally been deemphasized in all professions. Even child and youth care practitioners do not often recognize how important what children and youth are doing is to enhancing their ability to form relationships and to gain benefits from relationships.

While there are some writings on activity and activity programming in child and youth care (e.g., Barnes, 1991; Burns, 1993; Phelan, 2001; VanderVen, 1985; VanderVen, 1999), the daily reality of many children and youth is still fraught with boredom, lack of challenge and engagement, and efforts to overcontrol by adults that fail to take into account the effectiveness of activity involvement in mediating acting-out behavior. In essence, the best care settings may offer therapy and warm, caring, relationship-oriented staff, but not enough to *do*.

The stereotyped notion of activities is that they can keep children and youth "busy." Indeed they do, but it is a very productive type of busyness, if the activity is designed and conducted well. Among the areas of development encouraged by activities are the ability to plan, to take the perspective of others, to communicate, to develop skills that enable positive interactions, engagement with the wider world, and preparation for adulthood. Werner and Smith (1992) show that activity serves as a mediator for children and youth at risk and that those who are involved in productive activities are more resilient.

I contended (VanderVen, 1999) that the development of self is enhanced by the involvement of children and youth in activities within the context of relationships and showed how activities can help promote the development and maintenance of relationships. This made the point that relationships do not form or evolve in a vacuum. Relationships and the form and content of communication within these relationships are nurtured as people focus on an activity or interest and are shaped and extended by the context of these activities.

SOME RELEVANT IDEAS FOR A NEW CONCEPTUAL SCHEMA FOR ACTIVITY-ORIENTED FAMILY-FOCUSED CHILD AND YOUTH WORK

If we are intending to increase the role of child and youth workers in family-centered work utilizing a relational approach, then we can transfer the same premise about relationships and self-development as supported by activities to family-oriented work. The three streams described briefly above provide the core of this conceptualization.

However, there have been some interesting and innovative concepts in the child and youth work field over the past decade or so that, if introduced into the formulation, may make family-focused activity oriented practice even more powerfully conceived and effectively carried out.

This paper thus represents an initial effort to develop a conceptual schema for deriving practice premises for activity-oriented family-focused child and youth work using these various "streams of thought." Their description follows.

Cohort Effects

Cohort effects are results and events in a population living during a given time period that can be attributed to the particular nature of the times in which they are living. Among youth, for example, a certain behavior may be accounted for by considering it as a cohort phenomenon. Social change promotes a behavior and, thus taking place, it then becomes an option for others. For example, teenage suicide might be considered a cohort effect. With a few occurrences, it then becomes named. Once something is named and comes into public awareness, it then becomes an option.

For example, there has always been suicide, including teenage suicide, but in the last several decades, awareness of teenage suicide–and the suicides of younger children–has grown, along with associated intervention efforts.

In recent years, there have been cohort effects among parents. These include becoming parents at younger and younger ages and, due to various social and familial upheavals, these neophyte, youthful mothers and fathers becoming "unparented" parents (Jashinski, 1994). "Unparented" parents are expected to provide an attachment figure, care, nurturing and stimulation to their children without having ever experienced these on a consistent or healthy basis themselves. Obviously, this poses challenges to their ability to be supportive parents in all of the ways parents are expected to rear their children.

This has great implications for family-focused child and youth care work and for adding the activity dimension to it. Some consideration must be given to applying a similar approach, carefully adapted to the parents if we are to expect them to become more invested in and functional in their relationships with their children.

The Daily Life Space

While child and youth care was initially conceptualized as working with children and youth in their daily life space, as the field has evolved there has been some movement away from this core role as new roles evolved: family or program specialist, developmentalist, and many others. With family-focused work, I suggest we once again turn to the fundamental role of the worker in the daily life space with the children *and* with their families. This approach has been described by Garfat (2002). He points out that "Family life is lived in" daily events (p. 3), and in these daily events there are patterns of interacting. If the worker intends to influence these patterns, then the worker must do this work in those settings where the families live their lives, not in the artificiality of an office setting. Utilization of the actual place in which families live enables them to make and practice change in the context of their real life and attached to real events and observations rather than reports.

Life Space Interview

Durkin (1988) points out the power of the "life space" interview for developing interpersonal skills by using an immediate occurrence in the life space to review contributing factors, how it was viewed and handled, and alternative ways of viewing and handling it: an opportunity to gradually correct reality with the direct participation of those involved.

Because much activity can or should occur in the life space, the emphasis on the role of the worker in the life space will be to encourage family-oriented activity there.

Relating to the Relationship

Given the profound significance of relationship in development and in support of the movement towards relational child care, there are hidden considerations. Anglin (1984) points out that when working with a parent and child or a child and both parents, the worker might inadvertently relate more strongly to one party than another. If the worker focuses more on the child, as she or he might be accustomed to doing by reason of training and past experience, the parent is omitted and unhealthy dynamics can develop. Similar unproductive side effects can occur if the worker relates more to the parent than to the child or even if she relates equally well, but separately, to each. Thus, Anglin (1984) recommends that the task of the worker is to encourage a stronger bond between parent(s) and child than to himself and to then be able to *relate to the relationship*. In this way the worker can truly support the positive development of both parents and child. The worker's communications may refer to the interactions between the parent and child, and model positive ways of communicating they can use.

Oxygen Principle

On airplanes, we have all experienced the instruction that should pressure decrease and oxygen masks be indicated, parents should put their own masks on themselves before helping their children. Of course, this is counter-intuitive. Would we not want to help our children before ourselves? However, there is an important lesson here for our work with parents: *Before parents can truly accept and apply more nurturant and sensitive methods of parenting, they must first feel more nurtured and cared for themselves.* I have named this concept the "Oxygen Principle" because it is so well illustrated by the airplane example. Introducing activities to parents can be a safe and productive way of offering such direct nurturing and care. This might be done either by suggesting or encouraging an adult type activity that a parent might enjoy, or giving parents an opportunity to play with materials brought for their children before they are offered to the children.

Re-Parenting and De-Parenting

We must not only focus on nurturing and caring for our child clients but in family-focused work must prioritize nurturing parents and avoiding their exclusion or implicit or explicit criticism of them for "causing" their children's difficulties.

This is where Soth's (1986) powerful concepts of re-parenting and de-parenting are important. Soth bases her work on Franz Alexander's (cited in Soth, 1986) notion of the "corrective emotional experience which states that over a period of time emotionally charged attitudes developed in childhood will have to be corrected by reliving similar situations in the immediate presence" (p. 111). In re-parenting workers recreate a nurturing and caring experience that makes up for gaps and lacks in a child's–or parent's–earlier experience. In de-parenting, dysfunctional learning about relationship that may have occurred in the context of a family are addressed by showing new ways and allowing them to be experienced and practiced in the life space. We can thus consider how we can use the de-parenting and re-parenting notions not only with children but also with their parents.

Incidentally, this is another rationale for why family work in the life space can be so effective. It enables workers to show caring and support by the very fact of "going to the family" rather than having the family come to them (Garfat, 2002).

Rhythmicity, Synchronicity, and Presence

While there has been a great deal of attention in the developmental literature to such factors as attachment in relationship formation, there has been much less attention to important related components that have been highlighted in the child care and developmental psychology fields. These are rhythmicity (Maier, 1992), and other transactional interactions that enable connections to be made in energy flows between people and for meaningful relationships to be formed. This process is akin to a "dance" of shifting movements (Krueger, 1999). As Carol Gilligan (2002) put it, "The experience of relationship [is] being in sync with another person" (p. 9). To these notions Krueger (1999) adds that of "presence," referring to the dynamic interactions between people and a task.

If rhythmicity, synchronicity, and presence are the key features of positive relationships and interactions, and presence is enhanced in the context of a "task at hand," then activities may serve to encourage and enhance these phenomena in family-focused work.

Primary or Key Workers and Multiple Caretakers

As with the re-parenting and de-parenting constructs, human service professionals have tried to conceptualize familial type approaches to group care. One such approach is the "primary caretaker" model (McElroy, 1988). In this model child and youth workers, rather than relating peripherally to a large number of children, are assigned a much smaller number for whom they serve as a primary caretaker. The role includes providing more individual attention and support in a relationship and serving as the coordinator of the more specialized services and experiences in the child's life. A counterpart model is that of multiple caretakers and the positive role these can play in the lives of children and youth in group care. Schneider-Munoz (1996) shows us how a multiple caretaker model, in which youth needs for a primary relationship change over time as the youth changes, can be very effective. Some youth, especially in the initial stages of group care, may actually best handle multiple caretakers rather than a primary caretaker. Multiple caretakers enable the avoidance of premature closeness or familial-type relationships that a child cannot yet handle and "distributes" responses to challenging behaviors among several people, lessening their threat. At different times, workers, employing their own styles and background, provide love, strong limits, structure, activities, and a trusting background for contesting the rules and participating in decisions.

A combination of the primary caretaker and multiple caretaker roles is feasible in child and youth care work with families; and integrating activity into the interaction can provide a context for applying these different approaches as indicated. Activities can be very neutral, focusing on a skill and product, such as doing a numbered painting in careful sequence, at some distance. They can also be programmed to encourage closeness, such as making pictures or collages of the family itself.

IMPLEMENTING ACTIVITY-ORIENTED FAMILY-FOCUSED CHILD AND YOUTH CARE WORK

The following is a pragmatic consideration of how the concepts already presented might be applied in activities.

Culture of Childhood

The "culture of childhood" refers to that array of specialized lore, knowledge, and skills that are endemic to children themselves and are particularly understood by children (VanderVen, 1996). For example, we all know how to make "fortune tellers" out of paper, wherever we were brought up. That is a piece of "lore" conveyed through the "culture of childhood" in a process of transmission across geographical lines from child to child. "Culture of childhood" activities serve as a means for children to make connections with each other and to engage in mutually known activities. The "culture of childhood" may be considered the "social coin" of children. They carry it with them wherever they go and that enables them entry to other child groups.

Regrettably, children and youth "at risk" and those who have experienced various gaps in their upbringing, for whatever reason may not have had the opportunity for interaction with their peers in normal environments that enable them to learn the activities of the "culture of childhood." This suggests that *adults* must teach these activities. If due to cohort effects parents do not know them, then child and youth workers must convey them perhaps first to parents and then encourage parents to share them with their children.

Meta-Messages

To provide or encourage an activity in family work offers a meta-message of "giving." A conversation in which a person is given the undivided attention of someone else certainly can make the recipient feel valued. However, when there is a chosen activity as the context in which the conversation takes place, that can make the participant feel even more attended to and cared for. There is not only the decontextualized interaction among parties but the perception that they have been offered something that is stimulating, fun, gratifying, and perhaps useful for the future.

Life Space Activity Programming, Recreation, and Office Sessions

In some group care, residential, and treatment settings, activity programming is delivered by a formal "Department of Recreation." Certainly these organized and planned activities are a core part of the children's program. However, where "Recreation" departments are stretched and clients have "recreation" programs for short periods of time, say, 90 minutes twice a week, it is not enough to provide a sufficiently rich and stimulating program for the children. Thus, it is crucial to reiterate the importance of activity programming in the life space as the responsibility of child and child and youth care workers. What the children and youth do after school until bedtime and on weekends comes directly within their purview and involves providing activities. While some recreation departments have actually developed family-focused recreation programs (e.g., DeSalvatore & Rosen, 1986), certainly a laudatory contribution and a step forward, this is somewhat different from the "life space" utilization of activities I am advocating here. Similarly, counseling or office-based approaches that utilize play and activity to encourage relationships (e.g., Griff, 1999) are a step forward toward the life space approaches we are advocating here.

Experiential Teaching and the "Experience Arranger"

Phelan (2001) pointed out that activities serve to transform the traditional office-based approach to counseling, in which experiences are discussed out of context, into the reality of the daily life space of clients. They provide the opportunity for *physical experience* and encourage sensations that promote learning and encourage memory, thus providing a more fertile ground for discussion, review, retention, and application. Play and activity are ideal means for providing physical experiences that include also the rhythmicity that we earlier discussed as a significant component of relationships.

The role of the child and child and youth care worker, proposes Phelan, might be that of an *experience arranger*, that is, the worker uses activities and other experiences to provide a context for the clients to review their belief system and then change it in the light of new sensations and experiences.

Phelan's (2001) two notions of using activity as a means of experiential teaching in which activities serve as the framework in which teaching and reflection can take place, and the child and youth worker as experience arranger, have implications for adding that role into activity-oriented family-focused child and youth care work.

TOWARD ACTIVITY-ORIENTED FAMILY-FOCUSED CHILD AND YOUTH CARE WORK: THE STREAMS CONVERGE INTO A RIVER OF PROGRESS

Given the fundamental streams of family-focused work, relationships, activity programming, and the varied concepts that have been added to these, how then might activity-oriented family-focused care work? What would it "look like?"

Activity-oriented family-focused work builds on working in the life space of the child and his family, specifically, the home, neighborhood, and community. A worker making a home visit, for example, would be alert not only to the interactions and dynamics among the family members but also to the activity material: how the house is set up to provide areas for activities and play, what family members "do" together, and what situations promote dysfunctional interactions or acting out behavior of the children. There would be some recognition of the fact that many parents may not be supplying a suitable "play and activity diet" to their children because they have not experienced this themselves. Thus, the worker would try to find out what interests the parents might have had, or have now, that she or he can support, and then build on the parents' new interests and experiences to help them see how their offering of and setting up activities for their children can encourage much more positive be- havior and serve as the context for more harmonious parent-child interactions. For example, solving a jig-saw puzzle as a family might uncover important interactional patterns, and these might be much more constructive than those that emerged from children running lackadaisically around the house because there are no activities or activity materials to engage them, leading to the par- ents' scolding and yelling threats. Similarly, the puzzle solving and the inter- actions that surfaced could be used by the worker as a more benign way of having a life space interview, showing the family the patterns of communica- tion that they are using and modeling more constructive ones.

Utilization of activities can provide an ideal means for a worker to relate to the relationship between parents and children and strengthen it. Rather than taking a child to a museum, for example, thus relating to the child alone, the worker might suggest a museum outing to the family, perhaps to a children's museum where there is a variety of interactive exhibits that both adults and children can enjoy together. Or the worker might bring a game or craft project to the home. Rather than "doing" it with the child, or alone with the parent for that matter, the worker might show it to all family members and work with them to get it set up and properly underway.

A worker applying the "Oxygen Principle" might determine not only what the children are interested in as a way of encouraging relevant activities, but also what the parents are or have been interested in. They can be encouraged to develop and build on these interests. The parents can be helped to see that pur- suing a hobby or interest enhances parenting skills, because the parent be- comes a more salient resource for the child as well as a happier person. For example, Mr. Jones might say that he has always wanted to build model planes but never could as a child. The worker might go so far as to offer to go with him to a hobby shop to pick out a model to start with. Or Mrs. Reed may say that she always wanted to arrange flowers. This could initiate a discussion of start- ing a family flower garden, taking a flower arranging class, and the like. With the "meta-message" of giving offered by focusing on an activity, and the atten- tion directed at the parent with gaps in experience, the parent is strengthened as a person and thus as a parent. It can also be added that when the activity is in- troduced to and through a parent, there is less likely to be an unspoken jealousy of a parent towards a child who is being generously given an activity that the parent never had.

If we consider that a healthy family provides a good diet of play and activi- ties for the children, then activity is a key aspect of both "re-parenting" and "de-parenting." Some workers have had great success with parents in allowing them to experience traditional early childhood "hands on" activities: water play, finger painting, crayoning (drawing), collage, playing with sand and shaving cream, block building; in a sense providing "re-parenting" through these activities. Any number of activities can be employed to support "de-parenting": art, games, sports, and the like. Within the context of the activity, dysfunctional patterns of relationship become apparent. As mentioned before, these provide a richer and less threatening backdrop for the life space family "interviews" that point these out, how they are working, and how they might be changed. In fact the activities can also provide a framework for applying and practicing the changes: "The next time Jimmy keeps trying to put the wrong piece in when we are doing a puzzle," says Mr. Green, "I won't call him stupid. I remember when my father did that to me. Rather, I'll say, 'Why don't you try another place, like over here?'"

Almost all activities–if not all of them–automatically embrace the rhythmicity and synchronicity that we now recognize as a fundamental aspect of relationships. Playing catch, doing a puzzle, making and decorating cookies, finger painting, stitching up doll clothes, making a model plane, sawing a piece of wood–all have a rhythmicity and physicality. Doing these together, whether or not the parent is the facilitator or a joint participant, sets up the rhythmic component that can situate interaction and promote its synchronicity as well. The activity can serve as the focal point or task that encourages "presence" as described by Krueger (1999) to emerge.

Activities can support the array of care-taking roles, from primary to multiple–in a family-based approach. Like their children, parents may need to be engaged initially in a way that allows some productive distancing. Certainly a parent might feel less intruded upon if she or he is offered, for example, an intriguing wire puzzle to try, "just for fun," rather than a formal interview in which he is to discuss significant life events. As often happens when people interact more casually over an activity, there is such a heightened comfort level that personal revelations begin spontaneously to be offered. The selection and conduct of an activity can address the particular phase of ability to tolerate closeness. In general, more structured materials–such as tiles, craft sticks, board games, and the like enable some distancing while still providing a context for face-to-face interaction. More plastic media, such as paints, with less structure encourage expressiveness and revelation and hence might not be introduced until some comfort level and basic trust were established.

It is the very fact that people can so much more readily be reached when they are enjoying doing an activity together that supports the notion of activity-oriented family-focused work in the life space of home, yard, neighborhood, and community. This is different (although by no means better) than utilizing activities to enhance communications or to help reach specific goals in an office or formal recreation situation. In an ideal world, all would be available as a spectrum of client services.

The notion of the culture of childhood supports the idea of the child and youth worker having a bag of tricks (portable activity knowledge and skills) so as to share with parents or with a child who then teaches his parents. Adults who have not experienced such things as table top footballs, fortune tellers, paper airplanes, children's jokes–all of these features of normative culture of childhood–are amazingly engaged and intrigued when they have the permission of another adult to enjoy them. Such activities are one way of delivering a meta-message of caring.

Activities are an ideal means of experiential teaching, since their physical and rhythmic aspect encourages "muscle memory," provides something specific to reflect upon, and serves as a focal point for discussion of a situation or event. Activities also provide a context for practicing a new approach or skill in a concrete way. For example, if a worker is encouraging a parent to provide more positive guidance to a child by stating things affirmatively, for example, "Hold your sister's hand," rather than, "You'd better not let your sister go out in the street," having the parent engage the child in a new activity that the parent can lead provides an ideal arena for such practice. Here, the parent might work to say something like, "Place each stick on top of the other," rather than "Don't let them land every which way."

Assessing the role of activities in the lives of families, determining the resources they have for activities, selecting appropriate activities to promote established goals, using activities to develop and mediate relationships, and approaching and supporting parents and families through activities are all part of being an "experience arranger." These are all aspects of activity-oriented family-focused child and youth work. It could thus be feasible to consider what competencies workers need in order to do this work.

CONCLUSION

The vignettes that opened this paper were selected to show how an activity-oriented family-focused approach could address the common issues illustrated. Let's look at them again in the light of what has been presented in this paper.

The first incident, with the bored youth acting out until they were deprived of their home visits, would be less likely to happen in a program using a family-centered model in which good behavior is not matched with family contact and in which a rich activity program would at least partially address the complaint of boredom.

In the second vignette, Mrs. Smith laments how her son lies around with "nothing to do." The door of course is open for an activity approach that offers

Mrs. Smith experiences and resources that she can use with her son as well as some that directly engage him in productive activities that offer him experiences that he can then discuss with his mother. For example, the worker might bring an array of games and set them up so mother and son play together with the worker cheering them on. When the son has developed the skills of a game, both worker and mother can support him in playing it with peers. The worker can help the mother find community activity resources for her son, such as after school clubs and community sports.

Josie's mother, who has received so little nurturance herself as she tries to deal with everyone else's problems, needs a bit of "re-parenting" and some pleasant, engaging experiences. In a family-focused activity-oriented approach, the worker would be trying to find out what might interest this mother in terms of an activity for *herself*. Perhaps she has always wanted to draw and paint. The worker could help her join a class, possibly. With her own investment in an activity, she would then have a base for recognizing the importance of similar activities for her children.

The counselor trying to set up a reward system sounds so technical and removed from the reality of daily living of the family in his office that he loses their attention (not of course to speak of the fact that the approach is questionable in the context of effective utilization of activities). A home visit, in which the worker observes Joey's behavior, the family's responses, the resources available to Joey and the family, works with the family to experience for both themselves and Joey an array of interesting and engaging activities might bring quite different results.

The field of child and youth work has made tremendous strides in scope and definition in recent decades. From a sole focus on children and youth it has moved into a more ecological, contextual approach in delivering its special services to families. The field has pioneered an array of concepts that can be "re-cycled" now to enhance its contribution to promoting positive family, parent, and child and youth development.

REFERENCES

Ainsworth, F. (1997). *Family centred group care: model building.* Brookfield, USA: Ashgate.

Anglin, J. P. (1984). Counseling a single parent and child: functional and dysfunctional patterns of communication. *Journal of Child Care, 2*(2), 33-45.

Barnes, H. (1991). *From warehouse to greenhouse. Play, work and the routines of daily living in groups as the core of milieu treatment.* In J. Beker, & Z. Eisikovits (Eds.), *Knowledge utilization in residential child and youth care practice* (pp. 123-156). Washington, DC: Child Welfare League of America.

Burns, M. (1993). *Time in.* Sarnia, Ontario: Burns and Johnston Publishing.

DeSalvatore, G., & Rosenman, D. (1986). The parent-child activity group: using activities to work with children and their families in residential treatment. *Child Care Quarterly, 15*(4), 213-222.

Durkin, R. (1988) "Therapeutic" child care: a competency-oriented interpersonal approach. *Child and Youth Care, 17*(3), 169-183.

Fewster, G. (1990). Growing together: the personal relationship in child and youth care. In J. Anglin, C. Denholm, R. Ferguson, & A. Pence (Eds.), *Perspectives in professional child and youth care* (pp. 25-40). New York: The Haworth Press, Inc.

Garfat, T. (1998). The effective child and youth care intervention: a phenomenological inquiry. *Journal of Child and Youth Care, 12*(1/2).

Garfat, T. (2002). Working with families: using daily life events to facilitate change: A child and youth care approach. Unpublished manuscript.

Gilligan, C. (2002). *The birth of pleasure.* New York: Knopf.

Goleman, D. (1995). *Emotional intelligence.* New York: Bantam Books.

Griff, M. (1999). Intergenerational play therapy: the influence of grandparents in family systems. In V. Kuehne (Ed.), *Intergenerational programs: understanding what we have created* (pp. 63-76). New York: The Haworth Press, Inc.

Harter, S. (1999). *The construction of self: a developmental perspective.* New York: The Guilford Press.

Krueger, M. (1998). *Interactive youth care work.* Washington, DC: Child Welfare League of America.

Krueger, M. (1999). Presence as dance in work *with* youth. *Journal of Child and Youth Care, 13*(2), 59-71.

Jashinski, C. (1994). The "uncaring" or "unparented" parent: implications for practice. Unpublished manuscript.

Maier, H. (1987). *Developmental group care of children and youth: concepts and practice.* New York: The Haworth Press, Inc.

Maier, H. (1992). Rhythmicity–A powerful force for experiencing unity and cosmic connections. *Journal of Child and Youth Care Work, 8,* 7-13.

Mattingly, M., Stuart C., & VanderVen, K. (2001). *The North American child and youth care certification project.* (http://www.acycp.org) Association for Child and Youth Care Practice.

McElroy, J. (1988). The primary caretaker model: a developmental model for the milieu of children and adolescents. In R. Small, & F. Alwon (Eds.), *Challenging the limits of care* (pp. 29-43). Needham, MA: Trieschman Center/Walker School.

Phelan, J. (2001). Experiential counseling and the practitioner. *Journal of Child and Youth Care Work, 15/16,* 256-263.

Schneider-Munoz, A. (1996). Socially constructed worlds of high risk youth in the U.S.: a developmental and cultural case study of relationships in youth work. *Journal of Child and Youth Care Work, 11,* 72-83.

Selman, R., Watts, C., & Schultz, L. (1997). *Fostering friendship: pair therapy for treatment and prevention.* New York: Aldine de Gruyter.

Soth, N. (1986) Reparenting and deparenting as a paradigm for psychiatric residential treatment. *Child Care Quarterly, 15*(2), 110-120.

VanderVen, K. (1985). Activity programming: its developmental and therapeutic role in group care. In L. Fulcher, & F. Ainsworth (Eds.), *Group care practice with children.* London: Tavistock.

VanderVen, K. (1996). Towards socialization and harmonious cross-cultural relationships: integrating cultural universals and cultural specifics through activities of the "Culture of Childhood." Paper presented at the symposium, "The Many Cultures of Childhood." Cambridge, MA: Harvard Graduate School of Education.

VanderVen, K. (1988). Working with families: expanded roles for child care practitioners. *Family perspectives in child and youth services, 11*(1), 149-175.

VanderVen, K. (1991). Working with families of youths in residential settings. In J. Beker, & Z. Eisikovits (Eds.), *Knowledge utilization in residential child and youth care practice*. Washington, DC: Child Welfare League of America.

VanderVen, K. (1999). You are what you do and become what you've done: the role of activity in development of self. *Journal of Child and Youth Care, 13*(2), 133-147.

VanderVen, K., & Stuck, E. (1996). Model for agency and child and child and youth care worker preparation for family centered residential programs. In D. Braziel (Ed.), *Family-focused practice in out-of-home-care* (pp. 117-128). Washington, DC: Child Welfare League of America.

Werner, E., & Smith, R. (1992). *Overcoming the odds: high risk children from birth to adulthood*. Ithaca, NY: Cornell University Press.

What About the Dads?
Issues and Possibilities of Working
with Men from a Child
and Youth Care Perspective

Mark Smith

SUMMARY. The importance of fathers in their children's upbringing is increasingly recognised in child and youth care practice. Yet professional interventions in families often focus on men as problems. The experiences of fathers in community settings are applied to a child and youth care context. Workers are challenged to consider the role fathers play in their children's lives and how CYC principles might provide a basis for including men in their thinking about their work with children, youth, and their families. *[Article copies available for a fee from The Haworth Document Delivery Service: 1-800-HAWORTH. E-mail address: <docdelivery@ haworthpress.com> Website: <http://www.HaworthPress.com> © 2003 by The Haworth Press, Inc. All rights reserved.]*

KEYWORDS. Youthwork with families, youth care work, social work with families, family-centered residential care, child and youth care, family services, family support, parent education, residential care work and families

A number of strands from my own experience inform this article. It draws upon but does not reflect my practice of twenty years working in residential

Mark Smith is affiliated with the University of Strathclyde.

[Haworth co-indexing entry note]: "What About the Dads? Issues and Possibilities of Working with Men from a Child and Youth Care Perspective." Smith, Mark. Co-published simultaneously in *Child & Youth Services* (The Haworth Press, Inc.) Vol. 25, No. 1/2, 2003, pp. 149-167; and: *A Child and Youth Care Approach to Working with Families* (ed: Thom Garfat) The Haworth Press, Inc., 2003, pp. 149-167. Single or multiple copies of this article are available for a fee from The Haworth Document Delivery Service [1-800-HAWORTH, 9:00 a.m. - 5:00 p.m. (EST). E-mail address: docdelivery@haworthpress.com].

child care in Scotland where, looking back, we failed to engage properly with families. One of the reasons for this was structural. As residential workers we tended to internalize assumptions that we did not do family work, that this was the role of social workers and somehow required the kind of training and knowledge that we believed they possessed and by implication we did not. There was also a persistent confusion between family work and family therapy and an erroneous belief that both required some esoteric knowledge of the inner complexities of family structures and dynamics. More recently, the dominance of the child protection agenda and the location of policies and procedures for this at the level of community-based social work teams has compounded the sense that families were an area of practice demanding particular skills and knowledge.

Of course none of this made sense experientially. Many residential workers engaged skillfully and confidently with families, building relationships and trust that were beyond the scope of so many of those thought to be the experts. The task they performed was not often recognised systematically, nor were the opportunities presented by the strength of relationships they established with families capitalized upon.

If we did not do families, we certainly did not do dads. Where they were featured at all in the families of children, they were generally shadowy figures who rarely attended meetings and, more often than not, made sure they were not at home when we called. In some cases, where children had experienced significant harm at the hands of their dads, there may have been good reason for them not to be involved. However, it can become too easy within the child protection discourse to vilify men and to attribute motives or blame. When a dad did assert a role in their child's life, their approach may have been inarticulate anger, eliciting fear and suspicion amongst the professionals: "What does he have to hide?"

In contrast to this history, throughout my practice in child and youth care I maintained an awareness of the need of children and youth for a strong male figure in their lives and for them to be presented with positive images of masculinity. This view would not be held universally in the profession. Considerations of gender in forums such as the discussion groups on CYC-NET[1] can be sidetracked to focus on the role of men in maintaining control in an establishment rather than on what men, by virtue of their gender, might offer to children and youth. Indeed, the paucity of male workers entering the profession is rightly a growing concern in some quarters (McElwee, 2001).

Most men working in child and youth care, I imagine, can recall the sense of connection between them and particular youth for whom they represented something of what a youth wanted from a father figure. Rightly or wrongly, we took on some of those projections. These dynamics might be especially pronounced at different ages and stages of our own lives and those of the children and youth, reflecting different phases of what we represent to one another. Adolescents in pursuit of the "Who am I?" question might particularly identify with or indeed reject a father figure on the staff group. Moreover, consciously or otherwise, our own experiences of being a father or being fathered, and the beliefs we hold as a result, edge into our relationships.

Much of what we offered to kids, in response to their projections of the father role onto us, was no doubt positive. Developmentally there is good reason to provide a mentoring role to adolescent boys in particular (Biddulph, 1997). The trouble was that, with little real thought as to what we were doing and why, we tended to assume those roles irrespective of wider family circumstances and often substituting for rather than a supplementing the position of the natural father.

Having made the move from practice to teaching residential child care in a university setting, I was asked to help out on research project commissioned by a community-based family support service. The organisers of the project had realized the need to support fathers in the parenting role, but early attempts to do so elicited little response from fathers in the area. We, therefore, set out to try and ascertain the views and experiences of fatherhood of local men and to consider the kind of supports they would welcome. The men's backgrounds were varied. Some were in settled relationships, others were single parents, and still others were involved in custody disputes with former partners. A couple fathers were experiencing parenthood a second time in reconstituted relationships. We also canvassed the views of schools and other local service providers as to how they perceived the issues facing fathers and how they worked with them. The findings were used as a basis for the development of a project to support men in the parenting role.

On completion of this report (Cavanagh & Smith, 2001) we were asked by another family support agency wanting to develop services for men to undertake a similar piece of work. This time we focussed on the experiences of young fathers (Smith & Cavanagh, 2002). Together, the studies involved in-depth interviews with 29 men. While most of those interviewed were fathers to younger children, what was striking was the strength and consistency of views expressed by men from a range of different experiences and circumstances about their hopes for their children and about the pressures of fatherhood. Many of these views can usefully be generalised to the situations of the fathers of youth with whom we work.

Their stories will be used to explore how child and youth care workers might begin to include working with dads more centrally within their work with families.

A CHANGING SOCIAL CONTEXT

Changes in United Kingdom (UK) society have led to a diffusion of traditional expectations for men and have forced a reappraisal of fathers' roles within families (Joseph Rowntree Foundation, 1999). Employment patterns are less predictable and social forces are more complex and this is manifested in a more fluid family composition. The political discourse of the 1990s on both sides of the Atlantic was to seek scapegoats for this challenge to conventional understandings of the family. Single mothers and absent dads took the brunt of the political and media vilification. The Child Support Agency was set up in the UK to ensure that absent dads were not allowed to shirk their financial responsibilities for their children, perpetuating an image of men as feckless "jack the lads" who fathered children and then forgot them.

Little of this reflects the reality of a situation in which 8 out of 10 fathers in the UK still live with all of their biological children, and only 13 percent do not live with any of their children. Of these non-resident dads, 7 of 10 remain in contact with their children, according to Burghes (cited in Daniel & Taylor, 2001). Thus most children can count on regular contact with their dads.

However, the situation is different for children with whom we work in child and youth care and who are involved in child protection. Of these children, only 38 percent live with both parents. Thirty-one percent live with a lone mother, 28 percent in reconstituted families, and 2 percent with lone dads. The figures for those still with both parents drops sharply over time as child protection proceedings continue (Daniel & Taylor, 2001).

Since the late 1990s, the broader policy direction of support for parenting has increasingly been recognised as a cornerstone of the Government's early intervention and social inclusion agendas. A recent study identified as many as 800 initiatives supporting parenting in Scotland (Henderson, 1999). Within this, however, services geared more specifically towards fathers are few and far between. Indeed, in the wider focus on parenting, one study classifies fathers within the category of parents with specific needs (Henderson, 1999).

Practice Questions

- Where are the dads of the children and youth you work with?
- What are their circumstances?

Men as "Other"

In addition to possible marginalisation in the research agenda and in wider debates around parenting, men can also find themselves objectified.

The legal system in Scotland still fails to afford men automatic rights and responsibilities for their children unless they were married to the child's mother at the time of the birth. This situation is reinforced when it comes to service delivery. The social work department, for instance, has a statutory duty to work with parents, and within these parameters mothers generally describe themselves as both the primary carer and also the legal carer (Cavanagh & Smith, 2001). Men also pointed to institutionalized presumptions by the legal profession and the Child Support Agency in respect to a man's role in parenting. According to one father, "When I go to sign on, I am always asked why I'm not working."

Such presumptions can be further reinforced by professional assumptions. In the past, psychoanalytic or attachment theories could perpetuate what Buckley (1997) calls the mothering syndrome. More recently, some feminist perspectives, which have been influential in social work in particular, at times appear to attribute many of society's ills such as domestic violence and child abuse to the expression of a "hegemonic masculinity" (Cowburn & Dominelli, 2001). The notion of hegemonic masculinity is that a man's concept of himself and of his role is constructed in relation to an image of masculinity based upon power and dominance, especially over women and children. Such discourses have been incorporated into a practice orientation that can act to exclude men to an extent that O'Hagan and Dillenburger (cited in Christie, 2001) described a "pervasive and endemic problem" (p. 31). It is a particular problem in child protection work where, for a variety of reasons, including at times a legitimate fear of male violence, men can be marginalised in the conduct of investigations and subsequent interventions (Buckley, 1997). This situation can have a number of effects, one of which may be to make men feel cornered and ignored. Their resultant inarticulate and aggressive responses may then be used as evidence to support stereotypical views. Another consequence may, in fact, be to allow men to evade their parenting responsibilities. Yet in some instances, interventions in families point to a failure of the professionals involved to appropriately engage with men rather than reflecting any more rounded assessment of a situation.

Liam was a fifteen-year-old lad whose father had been labelled as violent by the local social work office. As a consequence, Liam's contact with his mum and dad was severely restricted and services to his parents effectively withdrawn. Gerry, his keyworker in the unit, was a particularly skilled, confident, and engaging character. He made contact with the family, built a relationship with them in the course of a number of home visits and joint outings, coping along the way with episodes of dad's drunkenness. Because of Gerry's own sense of himself, he never encountered any violence or threat of it. It was quickly apparent in his "being with" assessment of the family situation that

Liam himself, a big and reasonably together 15-year-old lad, well able to handle or extricate himself if the need arose, was not at any risk of violence. Indeed, he felt a responsibility to be there to ensure that mum and dad's drinking was kept in check, and, perhaps, as a 15-year-old that was fine or, if not fine, at least understandable and something we needed to work with.

The projected fears in this case were those of the social worker and at a structural level, the department's response to a notion of male aggression. As a result, Liam was denied access to where he wanted to be. Yet within a few months, Gerry had him back living at home, probably not in a manner that sat comfortably with our own middle class notions of what family life should be, but happy enough to be there.

This was a dad, upon whom all sorts of negative professional labels had been hung. Yet when engaged by a skilled youth care worker, it was apparent that like most dads, he had a love and hopes for his son. He admittedly was not great at seeing them through but again there was something to work with.

The point of this is not to minimise male violence but to acknowledge that it is not immutable or pervasive and that there can be a context that might change and be more responsive to different workers in different roles. The marginalisation of men within professional discourses often does not reflect the reality, complexity, or indeed the capacity for change within their experiences. There is a need to acknowledge these realities and to see behind the labels. More recent approaches to working with men in social work, while holding into a feminist perspective, do in fact acknowledge the need to work with them in order to help them change their patterns of behavior (Cavanagh & Cree, 1996).

Practice Question

• What assumptions do you make (about fathers that might influence your practice with them?

The Importance of Fathers

Whilst professional practice and many of the assumptions on which it is based fail to properly engage with men, there is an increasing recognition of the role dads play in child rearing (Lamb, 1997). Burgess (1997) describes a range of benefits to children of positive paternal involvement in families, including better educational achievement. A boy's distance from his father can cause or aggravate any behavioral problems he might display (Pleck, 1996). Indeed, the importance of men in raising boys is seen to be important in the growing literature highlighting concern about the difficulties growing up faced by boys (e.g., Biddulph, 1997; Gurian, 1999; Pollack, 1999). The symbolic importance of fatherhood is also acknowledged (e.g., McKeown, Ferguson, & Rooney, 1997). This may be particularly important during adolescence when children will need a realistic image of their dad to come to terms with their own identity (Daniel & Taylor, 2001). The intergenerational dimension emerged powerfully in our own research. These men stressed the importance of their own fathers, however imperfect they might have been, in facilitating their rites of passage to adulthood (Cavanagh & Smith, 2001). Several of the young men in our second study in particular defined their approach to fatherhood in contrast to their own experiences of being fathered. The hope of one was "To be a better dad than my own." Another said, "Didn't want to be like my dad and didn't want to get married because it just caused upset and unhappiness." He said relationships were about using people, and it was better to use and not get hurt rather than trust anyone.

A strong message is that young men need to be provided with positive yet realistic images of what it is to be a dad. For many of those interviewed, the images they did have were based upon negative impressions of their own experiences growing up. The oft-repeated desire to be a better dad than their own may be laudable, but it may not have much substance to it unless based on real rather than idealized alternatives.

Practice Questions

- What role did your own dad play in your upbringing?
- What role do you play in your children's lives?

MEN AS DADS

All of the men we interviewed expressed a strong desire to be good dads and could give examples of the kind of everyday activities such as bathing and storytelling they do with their children. Several looked forward to getting home from work to spend time with their kids. Fatherhood went beyond material and practical provision to "thinking about the kids and carrying them in your head." Providing a good and happy home was another key theme.

There was very little evidence in the interviews of authoritarian or disciplinarian parenting styles. Indeed, many of the men interviewed explicitly eschewed such approaches, often in reaction to their own negative experiences growing up. Any virtues that smacking might have were rarely extolled, although many could acknowledge that they did resort to it on occasion in response to their own frustration, anxiety, or sheer desperation.

The ability of men to fulfil the parenting role was also acknowledged by the young mothers we interviewed for the second study. There was an appreciation that difficulties in their own relationships need not detract from a man's ability as a dad. One of the young mothers describes her child's father as "one crap boyfriend but one brilliant dad."

The aspiration of men to be good dads is not always the image we associate with the dads with whom we work. I began to question whether the small sample we interviewed was representative, even if it did include a number of young men who had been in or on the verges of trouble growing up. Coincidentally, in the course of writing up the report, I bumped into a couple of lads I had worked with, 19-year-old twin brothers, both of whom had been through the whole range of care provision, including secure accommodation. Both had fathered a child. When I told them what I was working on, they were keen to talk to me. One of them told me his child lived with her mother around 150 miles away. I asked if he missed her. He looked at me with evident disdain and said, "Of course I do."

This perhaps should not be that surprising. The desire to be a father is a powerful one, and one not just based on satisfying a sexual need or a primitive drive to procreate. We recognise the strength of this pull when we think about young mothers but can be unaware of or underplay it with dads. Yet young men "go through the same emotional struggle and confusion that young mothers do. Teenage fathers often want babies as much as teenage mothers do, for many of the same reasons," according to the American Psychological Association (cited in Rolph, 1999, p. 63). Daniel and Taylor's (2001) research shows that young dads want to be included in their children's upbringing, particularly as good role models. The emotional pull toward fatherhood is further exemplified in the experiences of birth fathers whose children have been given up for adoption. One man described a sense of physical loss for a child given up at birth: "There is not a day goes by when I don't think of him. I feel as if there is something inside me that has been ripped out and I feel empty and nothing is going to fill that" (Clapton, 2001, p. 57).

All of this would suggest that men, by and large, do want to be involved in their children's lives and that that urge remains throughout their lives irrespective of their level of involvement.

Practice Question

• What hopes might the dads of the youth you work with have for their children?

Men Coping

Professional images of men as exemplars of a hegemonic masculinity were rarely apparent in the interviews we carried out. What was evident was a range of different experiences and different expressions of masculinity that were raw, often unremitting, and at times poignant.

One area that affected a number of dads was their confidence. Many felt that they would be better dads if they were working. It would provide more money but would also give them a status that they felt they had lost, particularly if their partner worked. The breadwinner culture was still strong amongst all ages interviewed, yet over two-thirds of the men in our first study were unemployed because of illness or disability or by being the sole carer for their children.

All men found that parenting could get on top of them, and whilst there were individual reasons for pressures, there were some common themes. Those dads in the main carer role found it difficult to cope with what they saw as constant demands for attention and felt they were "running out of ideas" to keep their children occupied. Arguments between children drained their energy and confidence. A number of them said they would often lose their temper and shout at the children. Men trying to find work found being around the house difficult. For those who worked it was often an experience of long hours with little return. Two dads in relationships each clocked up 129 hours per week on a regular basis as security guards. Another had to try and keep a small business on the side to fulfill his financial responsibilities for children in two different relationships. All of this severely limited the time they had to spend with their children. The partner of one of these men further restricted the time he was able to spend with his daughter, again casting doubt on images of a dominant masculinity. Those men with a disability felt frustrated that they could not do the things that "normal" dads do: "I can't even roll about the floor, far less take her for a walk. I feel that I am just lying here watching her life go by." For dads who were primary carers the fear of falling ill was a constant pressure.

A number of dads had no informal supports and were unwilling to seek help. The absence of regular adult company is a difficulty for men in the fathering role. One admitted there were times he would "sit down and greet (cry)." One man referred to regular visits to his mother as a godsend: "Even though she's a bit flaky, it's someone to talk to rather than always kids' stuff." Relationship break-ups were seen as a major pressure, particularly in attempting to insulate their children from the effects. Lone dads also found it more difficult than it had been previously, to sustain friendships after their circumstances changed.

Practice Question

- What difficulties and pressures face the dads of the youth with whom you work?

Dealing with the Pressures

Many men said they had little time for spare-time interests to help them relax. Some worked long hours which left them little time to see their children, much less take up hobbies. For dads who had spare time their activities were mostly house-based, solitary pursuits. Most of the men interviewed claimed they did not use alcohol and drugs to relieve pressures. They gave a number of reasons why they did not use alcohol and drugs. One was money. Another was the need to maintain control; alcohol and drug misuse could result in loss of custody or contact. In addition, a number of men had grown up in an alcohol-fueled violent home and did not want to pass this experience on to their own children.

All the men interviewed "bottled up" the pressures. Almost half of them felt they had no one to talk to when things were getting on top of them. A number of them were reluctant to talk to professionals, especially social workers, fearful of being regarded as not coping and of losing their children. Others saw themselves as self-contained individuals who should be able to deal with things themselves. Two men from ethnic minority communities were brought up in strict households that would not allow the discussion of their problems with others. Those with informal and family support living close by had regular contact but would not talk about emotional issues. "I would talk for hours about anything rather than what is going on for me with the kids and her." The fear of dads about exposing themselves as failures was a strong theme.

Yet carrying the pressure takes its toll. One lone dad stated, "I guess I am gonna' explode soon–can't keep all this in my head." Of the sample interviewed for the first study, 20 percent were diagnosed with depression and another one-fifth stated that they constantly felt depressed. This is consistent with more general concerns about the emotional health of men.

One of the young dads cast an interesting light on why men might not be as involved in their children's lives as they might be. He recounted his own experience: "They (the mother's parents) want her to stick in at college–get a decent job–they see me as a waster–not good enough for her. I'm starting to feel they are right and maybe I should just drift off the scene." This was a lad who felt a responsibility to his child and indeed to his former partner but was unable to negotiate a role for himself. His sense of just drifting away was a symptom of despair rather than evidence of irresponsibility. It is not difficult to imagine that many of the dads of the youth we work with may "just drift off the scene" not knowing how to assert and maintain a place in their kids' lives.

Practice Question:

- How do the dads of the youth you work with deal with the pressures they are faced with?
- Why might some dads not figure in their children's lives?

Services for Men

There was a persistent perception among men that services to support parenting cater to women. This was most strongly felt by those men who did not have custody of their children and only occasional contact. They said they wanted help to be a better dad but that it was difficult without regular contact and there was nowhere for them to get "training in being a dad." They believed there were a lot of local projects for women where the emphasis was on supporting mothers. The men did not object to this approach but felt they had been left behind and that there was "little advice and support for dads." One respondent referred to the advertising of services as "useless and not directed to men and dads."

The majority of men who access children's centers and nurseries felt uncomfortable because services were so "women dominated." This was a common criticism in terms of staff but also in terms of community space. In one children's center there are a large number of mothers who regularly use the community room, and some dads were intimidated to enter "the women's room" and felt excluded from that resource. This finding is consistent with other research by Ghate, Shaw, and Hazel (2000) which indicates an almost unconscious but institutionalised discrimination against men in children's centers.

Most dads did not think the staff in agencies understood their situation or needs and felt awkward about approaching them. This was particularly true of social work, with some men feeling they would be judged as poor dads because they were asking for help. A couple of men felt that support from social workers was not forthcoming when they had requested it but that the response when it did come was to judge them for the very issues they had asked for help with at an earlier point. The issue of the credibility of the professionals involved was highlighted, with a couple of men comparing social workers unfavorably with the probation workers they had encountered growing up. Where the probation officers "knew the score," the men resented being told about parenting by what one described as "a middle-class woman do-gooder." Men commented that when statutory services were involved with their children, they wanted to deal with the mother. A number of men resented "being frozen out and treated as a bit part."

Almost all the men interviewed felt that having male workers in services would make them feel more comfortable and more likely to use local services.

A number of men observed that they wanted to relate to someone who knew what it was like to be a dad in what they perceived as a women's world. Male workers were few, yet the men interviewed who used a local children's center found the sole male worker there helpful. "I felt I could talk to him easily." For most of the men there was an absence of appropriate services as well as barriers to existing services. Almost all dads were seeking practical help and emotional support. "A place that you could drop into without being 'assessed' a failed dad but could get non-judgmental advice and support with practical stuff as well as 'head stuff.'"

Over one-half of all men said they would value advice and help with parenting in the widest sense but in a way that did not look down on them. Some lone dads wanted effective and flexible child care to assist with return to work and to get some time for themselves to re-establish friendships. Advice about custody, contact, and child support was identified as a crucial area by a number of dads. "Living in a world dominated by women and courts who always take her side" was how one dad put it.

Opportunities for men generally to express their emotions are often lacking. Some of this is undoubtedly a feature of Scottish male culture. However, some of it may also be structural in the sense that few places or opportunities are available for men to talk about their feelings. A number of those interviewed identified a need to do so and indeed did so with some candour and insight to the total strangers interviewing them. It may be that, were services available to dads on a similar basis to those offered to mothers, men might take more risks in talking about their feelings. One older man who looked after his grandchildren said, "I've been there, bottling it up playing the hard man; it takes lumps out of you, and I am past the age of worrying about losing face. It's good to get the other boys to talk about what's eating them, things like custody."

Only one of the twelve surveyed agencies with a role in supporting parenting reported having more men than women on their staff group, a ratio of 3 to 1. Another agency had an equal balance. Staff groups in the remaining ten were heavily skewed towards women, three of them reporting all female staff groups and others ratios of 1 to 10 or 1 to 11. The use of services was likewise skewed heavily towards women. Those agencies for which we are able to provide (or obtain) figures showing men's usage of their services gave percentages ranging from 5 to 12 percent of total usage. There are likely to be many reasons for these figures, one of which may simply be that those men in full-time employment are not in a position to take up many of the services.

Possible attitudinal and cultural factors contributing to the low usage of services by dads emerged in subsequent responses. One agency respondent indicated that men might potentially become involved in nursery trips, for example, but tended not to do so. Another that operated a parents group noted that "no father has ever shown an interest in attending." Another did not feel able within their existing resources to offer anything specifically for men, indicating that any services accessed by men would have to be within the framework of existing provision. This would suggest that men are unlikely to access services merely because they are there, because many of the characteristics of the service will institutionally discriminate against them. There is a need to more proactively consider dads in the provision of services.

Practice Questions

- How might your own agency act to exclude dads?
- How might it be more inclusive of dads?

WHAT MIGHT A CYC APPROACH OFFER TO DADS?

From the foregoing sections we might draw the following conclusions.

- Dads are important in their children's upbringing.
- Most men have a strong desire to be fathers and generally are motivated to be good ones.
- For a variety of reasons, men do not always fulfil as important a role in their children's lives as they would like to.
- Professional beliefs, assumptions, and ways of working can label men as problems in family situations.
- Existing services are rarely geared towards supporting dads and may in fact institutionally discriminate against them.
- Many men would welcome support that they perceive to be credible and non-stigmatising.

This situation provides a solid base from which to consider a child and youth care approach to working with dads. An attraction of such an approach is that it offers the prospect of shifting views of men as objects to viewing them as subjects in improving the life experiences of their kids. Most men want to be these subjects.

There is perhaps a greater potential for CYC workers to develop roles in working with families and with dads in particular than there is for social workers. The social work role with families is increasingly bound up in the statutory requirements of child protection. As such, the professional focus can be about monitoring and maintaining a less than satisfactory status quo with families. The social work role has become potentially and at times actually stigmatising of families, according to Higham (2001). A CYC approach by contrast proceeds from an orientation towards change as Thom Garfat highlights earlier in this volume.

The CYC approach moreover is about making connections, which involve workers using themselves to connect at a personal level with those they work with. The centrality of "self" and "self in action" approaches in the CYC tradition signifies one of the fundamental differences between CYC and social work where the professional role seems increasingly to be about carrying out certain discrete tasks and following procedures (Fewster, 1990). As such social work, as it has developed, can act to privilege system knowledge over self-knowledge. Indeed the importance of notions of "personal style" in working in a CYC context may be threatening to some workers as it makes it harder to hide behind the professional role and potentially exposes the success or otherwise of their interventions to an assessment of their own efficacy.

Workers in child and youth care settings have something of a head start in adopting "self" and relationship-based approaches to working with families. They do so on an everyday basis with the youth they work with. Paradoxically too, there may even be some advantage in their comparative lack of status and training as this may allow them to maintain a more authentic closeness to those they work with, less distorted by a particular professional lens. The literature in this area tells us the best workers are those who are closest to the backgrounds and understandings of those they work with (Fulcher, 2001). Residential workers in this respect fare better than social workers.

All of this provides a solid basis from which CYC workers might become involved with families.

Practice Question

- What features of your own "personal style" might you bring to working with dads?

PERSONAL STYLE IN WORKING WITH DADS

Working with dads calls for particular understandings of the way men understand and interact in the world. That might often be best done on a man-to-man basis. The views of the dads we interviewed certainly suggest that for many men that is the case. Like it or not, there is a "man code" that is shared with other men. Cultural considerations flavor how it might be decoded. In a Scottish context the code is often pretty unsophisticated. Rituals of encounter revolve around half a dozen words. The first of these is a greeting, either, "How's it gaun?" or simply, "Awright?" The response to this may be another "Awright" or "Aye" or "Naw." The worker has to negotiate this initial encounter and to then take the conversation into other non-threatening points of contact, perhaps picking up on environmental cues about what a man's interests may be or perhaps initiating a conversation around football. In Scottish culture it will be important to understand the profound religious and cultural nuances that surround affiliation to particular football teams. Other cultures will have their own artifacts through which meaning in interpersonal encounters is constructed and which, if understood, may provide a way in for workers to engage with individuals and families.

In engaging with men there is a need to see beyond the taciturn exterior that many present, especially perhaps as a defence against professionals they hold to be judging of them and of whom they are perhaps legitimately suspicious. Engagements around the professional role and its authority are likely to be less productive than those which start from a more routine encounter as the following example illustrates.

Mr. Granger was a gruff, heavy drinking Scot if ever there was one. The image we had of him was as an authoritarian, ne'er do well who spent his time in the pub while mum struggled to bring up four young kids. Pete, the eldest, was with us. We had organised a sponsored cycle run in aid of a couple of charities. Pete asked us if it was okay if his dad put a bottle in the local bar to collect donations towards our sponsored effort. We agreed and later went along to the ceremony in the pub to crack open the bottle. It called for us to take a step back from the professional role for a bit and to put aside judgements about the rightness or wrongness of a family whose interactions and relationships centred around the local pub. The fact that we went along to his local and shared a few beers with him brought our relationship with Mr. Granger onto a more authentic level and was formative in our subsequent contact with him. It called for a particular interpretation of the professional role, however, and one that is frowned upon in social work where there seems to be an increasing suspicion of strong personally based relationships.

The assertion of a role for men in working with dads does not detract from the role many women also play in this area. Annie, a former colleague of mine, is one of the best, most intuitive workers with families I have come across. She exudes directness and confidence and the image of a strong mother figure, which many men need and derive strength from. The trick is to recognise and tune into the different and complimentary roles men and women can play in engaging with families. This may call for a reappraisal of some of the roles we traditionally ascribe to men. For instance, how often do we try and ensure a male presence when we hear that a dad is visiting the unit and may cut up rough? Male workers can enter into family situations of this sort already cast in the role of "bouncer."

In order to reappraise prevailing attitudes, CYC workers need to include dads into their thinking about how they might work with families. An awareness of the importance of dads in children's lives is a good starting point, as is an appreciation of the different circumstances and experiences of dads and of the roles they might play in their kids' lives. Essentially men need to become subject rather than object in our understandings of how families operate. For this to happen we need to engage them at a personal and meaningful level.

Practice Questions

- What are the roles and expectations of the male staff in your setting?
- How might this affect approaches to working with dads?

Assessment

When CYC workers proceed from the basis of acknowledging the role dads might play in their kids' lives, the initial task becomes one of assessing what that role might be. Before trying to do so, workers need to realise that a minority of men may, in certain circumstances, be dangerous, and a consideration before proceeding to work with dads is to bear in mind the element of safety for both child and worker. In some respects, that risk assessment may only become apparent in the course of ongoing contact. The fact that a man might have abused his children in the past should not by itself exclude him from any future role in their lives. The nature and degree of risk will vary with age, stage, and circumstances. Yet professional labels and assumptions about the ingrained nature of masculinity and of abuse can persist and may in fact impede the belief in the possibility of change, which is central to a CYC approach.

The assessment then needs to center on the particular role a dad might play in his child's life. Daniel and Taylor (2001) offer the following typology:

- *As partner with the mother*–in this category, the worker needs to determine the different roles each parent assumes. This might include an assessment of whether the family is a traditional one in which dad provides and mum nurtures or whether child caring responsibilities are shared. It should also consider issues such as who takes on disciplining and how support mechanisms operate.
- *As an "alternative mother"*–where dads take on child care roles that society would generally ascribe to mothers. This might be in cases where dad is the sole carer or in other situations where there is merit in supporting dad to assume responsibilities that mum for whatever reason is unable to fulfil.
- *As a "luxury"*–in these cases dads might be described as being "good" with the kids or offering support to the mother. In reaching a view as to whether or how to intervene in such situations a worker might want to consider more closely exactly what dad does and the implications of this.

Some men can of course be good with the kids without taking sufficient responsibility for the more mundane aspects of the parenting task.
* *As contributing something unique*–such as being a role model. Given the predominance of adolescents and, in particular adolescent boys, in residential child care, this categorisation may take on a particular significance (pp. 62-65).

A fifth category to consider might be that of the *absent dad*. Irrespective of whether they are currently part of the family or have even had regular contact, workers should actively consider how they might include dads in their children's lives. The views of the men we interviewed would suggest that they still thought about their children and were interested in their wellbeing. Also, the likelihood is that adolescents are going to want and need a realistic picture of their dad. Yet how often do we explore with youth the importance of their feelings for or attachments to their dads?

Practice Question

* What role do the dads of the youth you care for play in the lives of their kids?

INTERVENTION

Once a worker has determined some idea of the role a dad might play in a family, they will be better placed to identify how any intervention might be most effective.

The experiences of dads interviewed would suggest that interventions should generally be of the "being with" or perhaps a "doing with" variety. One of the young dads we interviewed said he would welcome support, "Provided they weren't going to preach at me about happy families, but it was about handling real life hassle." He went on to describe his preferred supports as "Somewhere you could get advice without thinking you are failing, just because you ask a lot of things, especially relationship stuff." This young man probably did want to talk about but his ability to do so was likely to depend on him feeling that any worker offering support was practical, credible, and probably one with whom he had established some sort of relationship and trust. CYC workers might do well to bear such views in mind before giving advice or embarking on counselling.

The most productive interventions for CYC workers might be what Phelan (2001) calls "experiments with experience" whereby workers become involved in families to arrange activities in a way that might allow dads and other family members to reframe their experiences and to retell their stories from a different perspective. Thus, rather than trying to counsel a dad about the desirability of establishing or re-establishing a relationship with their adolescent son, the worker, from the basis of a relationship with the dad, might arrange to go along on a fishing trip or an outing to the pool hall with a dad and son. That way they might pick up the rhythm of a relationship and pace the nature and timing of subsequent contacts accordingly.

The only way Mr. Granger felt he could define a role for himself in Pete's life was to do so on his own territory, the pub. He would probably have loved to be able to go cycling with us. Perhaps the task in working with dads is to try and find those spaces and opportunities where we can step onto each others territories or find neutral spaces where we can connect from a basis of discovering how we as CYC workers can help dads be the kind of dads most of them would want to be.

CONCLUSION

This has been an exploratory consideration of some of the issues that can face fathers. The experiences of men in this role and the difficulties they often encounter from traditional services suggest that the adoption of a CYC approach to working with them holds out a number of possibilities. Our own dads, irrespective of the roles they played in our upbringing, shaped who we are. Those of us who are fathers know the emotional power involved in the role. Yet sometimes, in our work with children and youth, we do not acknowledge that they too have dads and either do not factor them into our work or worse, still actively exclude them from it. As the CYC task is increasingly conceptualized in relation to families, it would be wise to consider how we might include dads in this agenda.

NOTE

1. Child & Youth Care International <http://www.cyc-net.org>

REFERENCES

Biddulph, S. (1998). *Raising boys*. London: Thorsons.
Buckley, H. (1998). Filtering out fathers: the gendered nature of social work in child protection. *Irish Social Worker*, *(16)* 3.
Burgess, A. (1997). *Fatherhood reclaimed; the making of the modern father*. London: Vermillion.
Cavanagh, B., & Smith, M. (2001). *"Dad's the Word."* Edinburgh: Family Service Unit.
Cavanagh, K., & Cree, V. E. (Eds.) (1996). *Working with men; feminism and social work*. London: Routledge.
Christie, A. (Ed.) (1996). *Men and social work: theories and practices*. Basingstoke Palgrave.

Clapton, G. (2001). Birth fathers' lives after adoption. *Adoption and Fostering, 25*(4), 50-59.

Cowburn, M., & Dominelli, L. (2001). Masking hegemonic masculinity: reconstructing the paedophile as the dangerous stranger. *British Journal of Social Work, 31,* 399-414.

Daniel, B., & Taylor, D. (2001). *Engaging with fathers.* London: Jessica Kingsley Publishers.

Fewster, G. (1990). *Being in child care: a journey into self.* New York: The Haworth Press, Inc.

Fulcher, L. (2001). Differential assessment of residential group care for children and young people. *British Journal of Social Work, 31,* 417-435.

Ghate, D., Shaw, C., & Hazel, N. (2000). *Fathers and family centres: engaging fathers in preventative services.* York: Joseph Rowntree Foundation.

Gurian, M. (1999). *A fine young man: what parents, mentors and educators can do to shape adolescent boys into exceptional men.* New York: Jeremy P. Tarcher/Putman.

Henderson, S. (1999). *Supporting parenting in Scotland.* Social Work Research findings No. 33. Edinburgh: Scottish Executive.

Higham, P. (2001). Changing practice and an emerging social pedagogue paradigm in England: the role of the personal advisor. *Social Work in Europe, 8*(1), 21-31.

Joseph Rowntree Foundation. (1999, June). *Fathers, work and family life.* Findings Ref. 659. York: Author.

Lamb, M. E. (1997). Fathers and child development: an introductory overview and guide. In Lamb, M. E. (Ed.), *The role of the father in child development* (3rd ed., pp. 1-18). New York: John Wiley and Sons.

McElwee, N. (2001). Male practitioners in child and youth care: an endangered species? *CYC-online* Issue 27. Retrieved June 30, 2003, from http://www.cyc-net.org/cyc-online/cycol-0401-irishideas.html

McKeown, K., Ferguson, H., & Rooney, D. (1998). *Changing fathers? Fatherhood and family life in modern Ireland.* Cork: Collins.

O'Hagan, K., & Dillenburger, K, (1995). The abuse of children within child care work. In A. Christie (Ed.), *Men and social work theories and practices.* Buckingham Open University Press.

Phelan, J. (2001). Experiential counselling and the CYC practitioner. *Journal of Child and Youth Care Work, 15/16,* 256-263.

Pleck, J. H. (1996). Paternal involvement: levels, sources and consequences. In M. E. Lamb (Ed.), *The role of the father in child development.* New York: Wiley.

Pollack, W. (1999). *Real boys: rescuing our sons from the myths of boyhood.* New York: Henry Holt.

Rolf, J. (1999). *Young unemployed, unmarried . . . fathers talking.* Working with Men, 320 Commercial Way, London SE 15 1QN.

Smith, M., & Cavanagh, B. (2002). *Lads becoming dads.* Musselburgh: First Step.

The Development
of a Parent Support Group as a Means
# of Initiating Family Involvement
in a Residential Program

Heather Modlin

SUMMARY. Working with the families of children in residential care is critical to the success of the placement. For a variety of reasons, parents of adolescents in one residential setting were not receiving adequate services during placement. A parent support and education group was designed and implemented to provide opportunities for parents to access support, learn new parenting skills and, ultimately, optimize their relationships with their children. The responses of both parents and staff to this program were favorable. The group is now a regular component of the organization's range of services, and served as a springboard to enhance family involvement in other program areas. *[Article copies available for a fee from The Haworth Document Delivery Service: 1-800-HAWORTH. E-mail address: <docdelivery@haworthpress.com> Website: <http://www. HaworthPress.com> © 2003 by The Haworth Press, Inc. All rights reserved.]*

KEYWORDS. Youthwork with families, youth care work, social work with families, family-centered residential care, child and youth care, family services, family support, parent education, residential care work and families

---

Heather Modlin is affiliated with the St. Francis Foundation.

[Haworth co-indexing entry note]: "The Development of a Parent Support Group as a Means of Initiating Family Involvement in a Residential Program." Modlin, Heather. Co-published simultaneously in *Child & Youth Services* (The Haworth Press, Inc.) Vol. 25, No. 1/2, 2003, pp. 169-189; and: *A Child and Youth Care Approach to Working with Families* (ed: Thom Garfat) The Haworth Press, Inc., 2003, pp. 169-189. Single or multiple copies of this article are available for a fee from The Haworth Document Delivery Service [1-800-HAWORTH, 9:00 a.m. - 5:00 p.m. (EST). E-mail address: docdelivery@haworthpress.com].

The St. Francis Foundation is a nonprofit, community-based organization that operates seven distinct residential programs for adolescents in St. John's, Newfoundland, and Labrador, Canada. Six of these programs are for young people in the care of the Director of Child, Youth, and Family Services. These are a group home, two emergency placement units, a specialized individual living arrangement, a treatment program for young people with sexually intrusive behaviors, and an independence training program. The seventh is an open custody residential treatment program for young offenders.

The organization is staffed exclusively by youth-care workers, from front-line employees to the executive director.

The organization has expanded rapidly since 1992, when it operated a single group home. Prior to 1998, there was a dismal lack of services in the province for families with children in care. For the most part, parents had very little involvement in the placements of their children while in care, either in foster homes or residential programs, and did not receive significant support, education, or other resources either prior to the child going into care or during placement. Within the St. Francis Foundation, there was virtually no family involvement in any of the programs and no services offered to families while their children were placed with the organization. Given that "family support is both one of the best determiners of a child's success in residential treatment and the most important single factor in determining the child's post-discharge adaptation" (Anglin & Glossop, 1993, p. 268), it was imperative that family support and involvement be added as an integral component of the organization's programs.

WHY INVOLVE FAMILIES?

The need to increase the range of services provided to families in this province had been well documented prior to 1998 (Child Welfare League of America, 1992; Government of Newfoundland and Labrador, 1997; Select Committee on Children's Interests, 1996). In an evaluation of the Department of Social Services Child Protection Services conducted by the Child Welfare League of America in 1992, it was stated that, while the Child Welfare Policy Manual set out "a clear philosophical framework which reflects progressive social work practice" (p. 29) and advocated for the preservation of families and removal of the child from the home only when all other options had been exhausted, some parts of the manual were not clearly drafted and the manual was not, therefore, always followed in the manner intended. The evaluation further identified the lack of family preservation and support programs, such as the Homebuilders Program, as a major gap in services across the province. In fact, the only types of services available to families at that time were respite care, homemaker services, counseling, and community mental health programs.

While there had been a shift in thinking towards the inclusion of families in child welfare services over the past several years (see, for example, Garfat & McElwee, 2001), this ideology had not been translated into practice. If anything, the move towards a family preservation philosophy had a detrimental effect on children and families involved with the child welfare system. Children had been kept at home under the guise of "family preservation" but there had been no actual "preservation" services provided to the families. In reality, children were simply kept at home for longer periods of time, the problems magnified, the children became more disturbed, the parents became more frustrated and, eventually, when the behaviors of the children became so severe that they could no longer be ignored, they were removed and placed in care. While the preceding may be an oversimplification, it rang true in far too many cases and, unfortunately, still does.

Once the children were placed in care, most available services focused on "fixing" the child. This was evident at St. Francis, where parents were not viewed as recipients of the services provided. An examination of the organization's mission statement and philosophy clearly revealed that the emphasis was completely on the child; there was virtually no reference to parents or families. Goals and objectives of all programs were completely child-centered, and contact with families was essentially limited to arranging visits, attending case conferences, and sharing information. As stated by Anglin and Glossop (1993), "a narrow focus solely on the needs and experiences of children, or even on the parent/child relationship, will ignore a large set of parenting issues equally important for the positive functioning of the child" (p. 261). In this regard, our programs were certainly not operating at optimal effectiveness and the lack of parent involvement had, among other things, contributed to low numbers of children returning home from our programs. The example of Jamie, aged 16, illustrates this:

Jamie resided at the organization's group home for four years; he moved in shortly after his 12th birthday. Jamie had been in care since he was 7 years old and, prior to his placement in the group home, had resided in several foster homes. All of Jamie's previous placements had broken down due to the foster parents' inability to handle his ongoing aggressive behaviors. Upon placement in the group home, Jamie was very angry and resentful, particularly towards his mother whom he perceived as having abandoned and discarded him. Jamie's father was not involved in his life at the time of placement.

Jamie's relationship with his mother was very strained. While he maintained regular contact with her through phone calls and visits, he was often disrespectful and hostile, particularly if she did not give in to demands he placed on her. He also "punished" her by cutting off contact for long periods of time. Jamie's mother loved him, wanted to have a relationship with him, but did not have the skills to deal with his behaviors and had issues of her own that were unresolved.

Staff in the group home did very little work with Jamie's mother in the four years that Jamie was in the group home. Inadvertently, for the first few years they tended to side with Jamie and actually reinforced his view that his mother was responsible for all of his problems. Mom did not receive support or assistance from anyone else during that time, either; she had over 20 social workers during the four years, most of whom she never even met.

While Jamie made considerable strides during his placement at the group home, his relationship with his mother did not improve at all. This impacted several other areas in his life: his attitude towards and relationships with females, the excessive amount of anger he carries around, and his continued feelings of rejection and abandonment. Even worse, he should have moved from the group home long before he did, but he had nowhere to go. Jamie opted into voluntary, extended care at the age of 16 so he could continue to live at the group home. Currently, Jamie is a young adult who is completely estranged from his family. This is a sad example of a missed opportunity. Jamie's life today could be much different if we had only recognized the importance of working with the family.

The need for parent training and support while the child is in care is highlighted by Noble and Gibson (1994), who state that "parents must cope not only with the difficulties that contributed to the placement, but also with the problems that occur as a result of the placement: grief; fear; and stress" (p. 319). These emotions can precipitate a variety of responses in parents, including blocking the return of the child to the home or sabotaging the placement by forcing the child to choose between them and the caregivers.

The maintenance of the relationship between parent and child has been shown to lessen the effects of negative peer pressure (Garland, 1987), reduce the feelings of rootlessness, rejection, and isolation (Garfat, 1990) that are common among children in care, and have a positive effect on the behavior of children and their ability to adapt to being in care (Noble & Gibson, 1994). It also reduces the tendency of children in care to idealize the absent parents or develop irrational fears and feelings towards their parents; even sporadic contact provides children with an opportunity to maintain a realistic picture of their parents' strengths and limitations (Littner, 1975; Palmer, 1995).

Involving family members in the treatment process provides to the child "concrete evidence that staff and family are openly working together, decreasing the risks of manipulation and secrets" (Noble & Gibson, 1994, p. 317). It also reduces "competition" between parents and youth care staff, which can arise when youth care workers are perceived as filling the role of substitute parents (Garland, 1987; Littauer, 1980; VanderVen & Stuck, 1995). Furthermore, family involvement signals to both the child and the parents that the problems do not lie exclusively with the child and are family-based (Garfat, 1990). "Including family members suggests to them that they have an important role to play in the helping process. Because of their involvement they may see themselves as resources, rather than as failures or causes of problems" (Garfat, 1990, p. 129).

THE CHALLENGES OF INVOLVING FAMILIES

Since there are obviously great benefits to involving families in the treatment process, why has it been so slow to occur in many residential programs? Some of the factors that contributed to this problem in our organization included increased demands on the child welfare system coupled with a decrease in government funding, working in a system driven by crisis, lack of specialized training available with regard to involving families, and the lack of professional recognition of the field and the limited role that had been ascribed to youth care workers, by others and by ourselves.

Overshadowing all of the above, and certainly playing a major role in the continuation of the problem, was the fact that families can be difficult to work with. "Parents can be interruptive, they have other time commitments which limits which hours they can be involved, and they have needs of their own and other family members which drain staff" (Garland, 1987, p. 27). They can be hostile, uncooperative, inconsistent, and unpredictable (Garbarino, 1983; Littner, 1975; Noble & Gibson, 1984; Palmer, 1995). They are sometimes difficult to engage, reluctant or unable to communicate openly with staff, and distrustful of anyone involved with "the system." In many cases, they are hard to locate or completely disinterested in being involved in their children's lives.

Parents are frequently excluded from the residential experience out of a misguided attempt to give the children a "fresh start" (Palmer, 1995, p.103) and free them from the disruption and distress that can be caused by contact with the natural parents. Parental contact may result in "a temporary worsening of the child's behavior and functioning. The child may become quite tense prior to the visit and extremely upset and unhappy and difficult to handle after the visit" (Littner, 1975, p. 176). This distress can be confused with damage to children, while, in fact, it more likely reflects a "conflict of loyalties" (Palmer, 1995, p. 104) or separation feelings (Littner, 1995) and points to the need for increased rather than decreased family contact. Such thinking can be difficult when staff are faced with situations like the following:

Paul, age 14, has been in care since the age of two. From the time he was taken into care until the age of seven, he was caught in the "foster care drift" and bounced around from home to home. At seven, he was placed in a foster home in a small community where he remained until he was twelve. The placement broke down at that time due to his increasingly aggressive, possessive, and "bizarre" behaviors. He was placed in the psychiatric unit of the children's hospital for a full assessment. The results of the assessment revealed no psychiatric illness but did include a diagnosis of "attachment disorder." Paul was placed in the organization's group home.

Paul had no contact with his natural mother since he left home at two years old. After he had been living at the group home for approximately eight months, he initiated telephone contact with her. After this had been ongoing for awhile, always at his initiative, he requested a face-to-face visit. His mother indicated to her social worker that she was receptive to this. Since Paul's mother lived in a small community five hours away from the group home, Paul's keyworker accompanied him on the visit. Months of preparation took place prior to the actual visit. Plans were made for Paul to visit his former foster parents at the same time, since they resided in an adjoining community.

Paul's visit with his birth mother lasted for less than a day. She was attentive to him for a couple of hours and then switched her focus to "flirting" with his keyworker. She did not appear to have remembered the visit until Paul actually arrived and was quite concerned about it interfering with her darts tournament that evening. Paul asked to cut the visit short and spent an extra day at the home of his foster parents, where he was received with open arms.

It is situations like the one above that cause staff to cringe at the thought of working with parents. It is difficult for staff to be supportive of natural parents when they are aware of how the parent has contributed to the emotional damage of the child and, even more so, when that damaging behavior continues (Littner, 1975). Yet one reason that parents behave the way they do is because of the way we approach them. This is clearly documented by Garbarino (1983) who advocates for the "use of social support networks as a way to enhance professional helping" (p. 4) and change the way in which we, as professionals and parents, relate to each other.

Working with families requires a shift in the way we think (Noble & Gibson, 1994). Youth care staff cannot continue to perceive themselves as "rescuers" of the children from their troubled parents (Garland, 1987). This has been one of the impediments to providing services to families. It is difficult for youth care workers who have become attached to the children with whom they work to refrain from being critical and judgmental of parents.

"The institution of a family-centered model in a group or residential care program automatically increases complexity by introducing more elements in the delivery system" (VanderVen & Stuck, 1995, p. 14). This makes the job more complicated, increases the workload, and can more than double the number of individuals on the caseload. All of this can require a significant increase in financial expenditures of the organization (Noble & Gibson, 1994) and certainly serve as a further deterrent to implementing family-based services.

SOME POSSIBLE SOLUTIONS:
STRATEGIES FOR WORKING WITH PARENTS

The literature pertaining to the involvement of families in residential care clearly outlines several approaches, models, and programs that can be used to incorporate services for families into a residential program. These include involving parents as partners in the treatment process, providing opportunities for parents to become active participants in the daily life of the program, expecting parents to maintain responsibility for their child after placement, facilitating regular contact and home visits, and providing parent education and support (Garland, 1987). All of these methods can be used alone or in conjunction with each other to provide a comprehensive approach to family involvement.

The various ways of working with families can be divided into two distinct categories: those that involve families directly in the residential program and those that provide services such as support, education, or counseling to families outside of the program.

In the first category, "the primary input role for family members is as participants in the treatment process" (Garfat, 1990, p. 138). Garfat provides an excellent illustration of involving parents and he describes the process of utilizing the skills and strengths of parents as a means of including them directly in the program. A mother who can sing and play the guitar can provide entertainment and lessons once a week to the young people in the unit; a parent with a knack for carpentry can assist with household repairs and maintenance; other parents can take on such responsibilities as offering cooking lessons, teaching art, and reading bedtime stories.

Parental involvement can take other forms. Parents can be assigned specific responsibilities for their child while in care such as purchasing clothing, attending medical and other appointments, and assisting with homework. Parents can also work as partners with the staff in establishing rules or helping to solve their child's behavior problems (Jenson & Whittaker, 1987).

At Parsons Child and Family Center, family work is the responsibility of the child-care workers in the daily treatment milieu (Littauer, 1980). Families visit the cottage for varying periods of time, ranging from one afternoon a week to extended visits of several days. These visits provide opportunities for child care staff to complete assessments on the needs of the family, model effective parenting and communication skills, involve parents in program activities, and offer direct help to the parents in the form of nurturing, sharing frustrations, and offering feedback and suggestions.

Garland (1987) outlines several strategies for moving an agency into a model of family intervention. She recommends that it is necessary to "draw the family generation line so that the child care worker is a partner with the parent" (p. 27). Clear lines of communication must be established so that the children are not able to manipulate one party against the other and to clarify and correct any differences or misunderstandings. Parents must also become frequent, active participants in the program, not just visitors. "Parents must either accept the parental role or give it up so that other permanent arrangements for a family for the child can be made" (Garland, 1987, p. 27). Furthermore, parents can be encouraged to interact with other children in the placement, besides their own, and become involved in special projects. Child care workers and social workers can collaborate on visits to the family home and as co-therapists in counseling (Garland, 1987).

For several reasons, we did not initially focus on implementing any of the aforementioned models of family involvement. Our experience with families up to that point had been quite limited. Staff had not received any training or education about this type of work and were not thinking in family-centered terms. The organization's mission statement and philosophy needed to be revised and program goals and objectives changed to reflect the inclusion of families. While it was our intention to move in this direction, we decided it was more practical to begin by providing services to families outside of the residential programs.

THE BEGINNING:
DEVELOPMENT OF A PARENT SUPPORT AND EDUCATION GROUP

A logical way to introduce the concept of working with families was for us to implement a parent support and education group. There were several reasons that a parent group was considered as a starting point for family involvement. These included the positive effect of the group experience in sending the message to parents that they are not alone, helping them to handle "feelings of isolation, guilt, and despair while allowing them to discover unappreciated strengths with an opportunity to share these with others in need" (Anglin, 1985, p. 16), and providing an informal, flexible, and adaptable setting in which parents could learn. In a group setting, parents are provided with an opportunity to deal with their own unresolved needs and issues and receive nurturing and support from other group members and the facilitators.

Parents need to be nurtured along with their child; expecting parents "to be solely invested in their children, to place the children's needs primary, is usually unrealistic and an exercise in futility" (VanderVen & Stuck, 1995, p. 18). The need for social support has been well documented by Whittaker and Garbarino (1983) and it has been suggested that models of skill training that have been demonstrated to be effective will not work in the absence of social support. The virtues of parent groups are extolled by Webster et al. (1979); Peterson and Brown (1982); Grealish et al. (1989); Jenson and Whittaker (1987); Noble and Gibson (1994); and Garbarino (1983).

While there are various approaches to group work with parents, the literature reveals many common themes. According to Anglin (1985), "virtually all of the major objectives for parent groups address one or more of the following areas of personal development: *knowledge*: providing information; *skills*: assisting in the development of new ways of doing things; *attitudes*: clarifying, altering, or strengthening values and beliefs; *support*: providing encouragement, validation, and resources" (p. 16). The content of most groups is remarkably consistent and includes a focus on child development, communication, self-care and support, parenting skills, and discipline (Anglin, 1985; Bavelok, 1998; Jenson & Whittaker, 1987; Peterson & Brown, 1982).

In order to begin the process of working with families, a parent support/education program was developed. This was designed to introduce the concept of parent involvement to staff in a non-threatening manner, provide an opportunity for us to connect with parents in a meaningful way and, ultimately, serve as a springboard for further family involvement in our programs.

Moreover, the implementation of a parent group could be achieved by the organization without additional funding or resources and, if successful, provide us with a rationale to obtain increased funding for the specific purpose of becoming a family-centered program.

As stated previously, in order for parents to be able to respond effectively to the needs of their children, their own needs must first be met. Since most of the families with whom we worked were lacking an adequate social support network, one of our first tasks was to provide support for parents and increase their ability to access support in the community.

The goal of the group was to provide support and education to parents of young people residing in the organization's group home and emergency placement units so that they could optimize their relationships with their children. The objectives were as follows:

1. To create a support network for parents and increase their ability to access support from each other, the organization, and the community.
2. To increase parents' knowledge of child and adolescent development and basic parenting practices.
3. To increase parents' basic knowledge of effective disciplinary techniques and behavior management and decrease the use of ineffective techniques such as screaming, arguing, hitting, and passive avoidance.
4. To improve parents' basic communication skills and increase the occurrence of assertive communication.
5. To strengthen parents' relationships with their children as evidenced by an increase in positive interaction and verbal self-reports from parents and children.

The parent group was designed specifically for our particular clientele. The Nurturing Program for Parents and Adolescents (Bavelok, 1998) was the main source of material, but we did not use this program in its entirety, and we also utilized material and ideas gathered from other parenting programs. Grealish et al. (1989) stated that a group for parents of children in care should remain flexible and adaptable to the needs of the parents. To that end, although the topics of each group were pre-determined, the specific content and methods of delivery were decided week-to-week, based on feedback and suggestions from the group, their responsiveness to various activities and exercises, and so on. The group relied on the use of adult learning principles and utilized a variety of teaching techniques such as role plays, videos, small group exercises, and discussion. The use of written material was kept to a minimum, as it was expected that some parents may have difficulty with reading or writing. Opportunities to nurture parents and teach self-care skills and concepts were purposefully incorporated into each group.

Evaluation of all objectives was conducted informally through observation of parents at each group, by requesting ongoing feedback from parents, and from an open discussion at the last group meeting. Questions that were asked at the last group included:

What was particularly meaningful about one or more of the sessions? Why? What are the most important things you learned? Were there some things you learned that were helpful but that you couldn't use? Do you have any suggestions on how the group could be improved? What did you like? What did you not like? Would you recommend this group to other parents? Would you be interested in continuing in this group, without the facilitators, if we could provide the space?

The group was held in the basement apartment of one of the agency's emergency placement units. This apartment was not serving any other purpose and provided a warm, home-like atmosphere for the group. It contains a kitchen, which is useful for storing and serving refreshments.

As recommended by Grealish et al. (1989), we offered to provide transportation and child care to those parents who required it. Refreshments were provided at each group, during a 20-minute break, which also provided an opportunity for the parents to socialize. On occasion, parents offered to supply the refreshments and brought in snacks such as cookies and cakes.

OVERVIEW OF THE GROUP

The parent support/education groups took place over a period of 10 weeks. In the two weeks prior to the first meeting, we focused our effort on recruiting parents. This was, by far, the most difficult part of implementation.

In selecting parents, we considered all parents of young people who were residing at our group home and emergency placement units and some parents of young people who had left either of these units within the past year (these parents had been informed of the upcoming group while their children were with the organization and expressed an interest in becoming involved). After ruling out parents who lived more than one hour's drive away and those with serious mental illness or active drug and alcohol issues, we were left with ten parents to approach. Each parent was contacted at least three times by telephone to discuss the group, and the first phone call was followed up with a written invitation. Most parents were initially very reluctant to commit. After much dialogue and what often felt like very aggressive salesmanship, we were able to arrange face-to-face meetings with 7 of the 10 parents. During these meetings, we gave more detailed information about the group and answered questions from the parents.

At the initial meetings with parents, they were asked if they needed transportation to and from the meetings. All parents responded affirmatively and indicated that without transportation they would be unable to attend. With some creative juggling of shift schedules and a little extra funding for staffing and mileage costs, we were able to use some of our youth care staff as drivers. Parents were split up into geographical areas, and drivers picked them up in groups of two or three, dropped them off, and returned for them at the end to drive them home. While different drivers were used from week-to-week, some staff developed an interest in this task and regularly requested to be selected as a driver. Parents and drivers developed some interesting relationships, and parents expressed appreciation for the drivers during our last meeting.

Of the six parents who attended the first meeting, five were female and one was male. The male member received a significant amount of attention from the females and was praised considerably for his "courage" in joining. All six parents remained in the group consistently throughout its entirety. There were only three absences and these were due to illness.

Prior to the first meeting, facilitators participated in six hours of training on conducting groups. This was very useful and provided both facilitators with concrete information and strategies to use during the groups.

Facilitators met weekly to determine the content of each session, which was geared towards the needs of the parents and dependent on the outcome of previous sessions. It was obvious from the very beginning that the parents' needs would have to be addressed before we could move on to discussing the needs of their children, as noted by VanderVen and Stuck (1995). Parents brought so many of their own difficulties to the group that, for the first four sessions, their children were not mentioned except as a source of frustration. By session five, parents were starting to mention their children more in conversation and the focus of the group began to shift. By the end of the group, most parents began check-in by reporting on the progress of their children.

All sessions began with a check-in and ended with a check-out. At the first session, we allotted five minutes for check-in, but this was not nearly enough time. In the second session, we attempted to use an egg timer to limit the amount of time for each person at check-in in a misguided effort to keep people on time and prevent any one parent from monopolizing the group. The parents were very quick to express their disdain for this idea and indicated that everyone should be given as much time as they needed. In the words of one parent, "If someone had a hard week, they should be able to talk about it for as long as they want. That's why we're here." We put away the egg timer and adjusted our schedule accordingly. The parents used check-ins as an opportunity to share the events of their week and catch up on what was happening with others. This became a time when personal information was shared and parents were consistently caring and supportive of each other. By the last few sessions, it was not unusual for check-in to involve lots of tears, laughter, hugging, and holding hands.

Another regular feature of the meetings was a weekly "lottery." At the end of each group, before check-out, parents were given an opportunity to win a $20 gift certificate from a local restaurant or store. To keep this interesting, we varied the ways in which this contest could be won, from bingo to lucky numbers, lucky chairs, and so on. Feedback from parents indicated that they found this portion of the group fun and, of course, they liked winning. The lottery was not mentioned by them as an important component of the group, however, and did not appear to have had any impact on retention.

The focus of the first session was on establishing rapport, developing group rules, providing an overview of future activities, and completing confidentiality agreements and consent to participate forms. Topics of other sessions included community resources, praise and encouragement, communication skills, expressing feelings, negotiation, discipline, anger management, stress management, basic needs, and self-care. Most groups ended with a visualization and relaxation exercise.

From the first group onward, parents consistently reported that they found the group supportive. At the end of the session on community resources, parents indicated that they felt much more confident and knowledgeable than they had previously about being able to access support and resources from the community. One parent stated that she had received the most support ever from our organization itself, not only while her child was with us but in an aftercare capacity as well. Other parents in the group echoed this statement. Parents' comfort level in seeking support and assistance from the organization was evident in the way that they contacted the facilitators at their workplaces in between groups. The two parents who still had children residing at the organization's group home dramatically increased their amount of contact with me, the program coordinator, and the group home staff. Some parents exchanged phone numbers and maintained contact with each other outside of group. One parent invited the group to her house for dinner.

During session five, we had a small Christmas party, since it was our last group before Christmas holidays. The parents had suggested that we exchange gifts and set a $10 limit on the amount to be spent. We exchanged names, and everyone received a gift during the party. As one parent opened his present, which was a gift box containing mugs and specialty coffee, he said, "I didn't think anyone knew I was in the world. Now look at this–I feel like I've been touched by an angel." This example speaks to the supportive nature of the group.

Parents were informed from the beginning that the group was scheduled to run for a ten-week period of time. This appeared to cause a great deal of anxiety for parents, who began as early as session three to express their concerns about the group ending. Comments were consistently made during every check-out about how much the parents would miss the group, how valuable the group had become for them, and so on. Parents unanimously requested that the group be continued beyond the ten weeks. After much consideration, we decided to continue the group on a monthly basis. We also extended the group by one week, opting to have the graduation ceremony the week after the tenth group instead of during this group. We took all parents to a local restaurant for dinner to celebrate the end of group and give them participation certificates. This event was very successful, and all parents appeared to enjoy themselves immensely.

Unfortunately, only 2 of the 6 parents had children residing in one of the organization's units during the course of the group. This made it impossible to observe or assess parent-child interaction for four of the parents. For the two parents we could observe, it was reported by program staff that parents' interaction with their children, while in the presence of staff, was more positive and parents were less inclined to criticize or engage in power struggles with their children. It is difficult to determine, however, whether this is attributable to the group or to the increased efforts of group home staff in working with the parents. At any rate, there is a correlation between the two that will be discussed later.

All parents reported feeling more confident in this area, although three of the parents had limited contact with their children, who were not living at home, and, therefore, little opportunity to practice these skills. We advised them to practice with whomever they had contact and reiterated that these skills are not just applicable to the child placed in care. One parent, whose child returned home during the course of the group under unusual circumstances, stated that she knew what to do in terms of positive discipline but had trouble doing it and still lost control when she became angry. The other parents were very helpful in pointing out to her what she was doing "wrong" and offered suggestions, based on their own experiences, on how she could improve. By the last few weeks, this parent was proudly sharing examples of situations she had handled effectively. While these were very small examples and, by the parent's own admission, many problems still existed in the home, they were a sign of progress nonetheless.

During the group, we observed significant improvement in the area of assertive communication for all parents but one. Over the course of the group, parents became much more comfortable in expressing their feelings and providing feedback to others. Use of "I" statements increased. By session three, parents were starting to hold each other accountable with regard to time, language, interrupting, staying on topic, and so on. One parent, who had been quite passive in the first few sessions, became assertive in expressing herself. This delighted the other parents, who had been encouraging and supporting this transformation. The parent in question became increasingly more vocal as time went on, and appeared to bask in the praise of her fellow group members.

At the last session, we involved parents in a discussion of the group and solicited feedback on what worked, what did not, what we could improve, and so on. Responses were overwhelmingly positive. Parents stated that the group was very supportive, all topics were excellent, the format was good, and all activities were fun and interesting. Parents stated that they had learned a lot. Specific comments from parents included: "You won't get another group like this one." "There was nothing about the group that wasn't good." "You could be yourself, no one was afraid of what someone would think." "My anger is more in check now than it's ever been." "If you change anything about the group at all, the next one will suck." The only recommendation for improvement was to lengthen the program.

Although the results were inconclusive in some areas and it is difficult to completely assess the degree of learning that occurred for specific objectives, there is no disputing the supportive nature of the group and its role in providing parents with a social network. Given that these were parents who were historically reluctant to participate in any type of formalized parenting program and were generally distrustful and skeptical of all professionals involved with "the system," the fact that we were able to retain them for the duration of the group and have them asking for more is a good sign that something worked. As stated by Grealish et al. (1989), "the first criterion in evaluating the effectiveness of such a program is . . . attendance" (p. 58). The parent group, although in need of some revision and fine-tuning, did appear to fill a void and provided parents with a much needed social support network.

What was most striking about this group, for both facilitators, was the level of neediness and isolation experienced by these parents. Although we were aware of this going into the group, it was still an eye-opener to grasp the reality of these parents' situations. They were dealing with all of the same issues as their children and, in some ways, were in much worse shape. In many cases, parents had a lot of information about appropriate parenting practices, absorbed through years of child welfare intervention but were unable or unwilling to translate this knowledge into action. Until the parents' own needs could be met, it was impossible for them to look after the needs of their children. In our session on basic needs, parents stated that they did not know they had needs. When one participant discussed this concept with her social worker, he told her that her needs were not important, she should only be focused on her child's needs. Being exposed to parents in such an intense and intimate manner certainly led us to reevaluate our views and attitudes towards parents and to hold more realistic and obtainable expectations for them.

One thing the parents consistently raised was the inconsistency in approach by social workers from Child Welfare, particularly with regard to disciplinary issues. One parent talked about being told by one worker to use timeout for her son when he was acting-up, then a new worker told her that the child was too old for timeout, then yet another worker told her she should be using timeout. Many of these types of stories emerged. Parents were frustrated, confused, and often had reached the point where they just gave up trying anything new. This usually resulted in them being labeled uncooperative or resistant to intervention. As put forth by Garbarino (1983), it is often the manner in which we work with parents, and not the parents themselves, that causes the problems. Parents in the group indicated that they were pleased with the information we provided because it clarified some of their previous confusion and misunderstanding.

When these parents joined the group, their own issues were at the forefront. If we had jumped in with a set agenda and tried to force this on the group, we would certainly have lost them. This was experienced by Grealish et al. (1989) when they tried to implement a conventional parent group with a similar set of parents. By validating them and attending to their needs, we were able to build relationships and trust and bring parents to the point where they were open to learning new things and being challenged on their beliefs.

Being responsive to the needs of parents required changing the content of some of the sessions. As an example, we had originally planned to cover the topic of child development in session two. After the first session, it was obvious that the parents were nowhere near ready to absorb this material nor would it have held their interest. At that point, they were looking only for information related to their own situations or, in terms of their children, specific things that they could do to make things better. We changed session two to a discussion of self-care and community resources. This session was very productive and more in tune with what the parents wanted and needed from the group. Child development was never actually presented as a full topic; we instead looked for ways to weave bits and pieces of this information into other discussions. This seemed to work well and gave parents information that was relevant to them at the time it was presented.

The parent support/education group had a significant impact on the entire organization. Staff viewed the whole project with great interest and were very curious about the workings of the group. For Christmas, staff took the initiative to raise money for the parent group and offered to purchase presents for the parents to give to their children. This was greatly appreciated by the parents.

Further, those staff who served as drivers were given first-hand exposure to the group. On their way home, parents often continued to talk with the drivers about issues that had been discussed at group. In one instance, a parent told her driver about her son's Tourette's Syndrome. The next week, the driver took it upon himself to bring her some written information. The value of working with parents spread throughout the organization, and staff became much more receptive to the concept. At the group home, the process of enhancing family involvement was started and staff became much more active in working with parents. Having two of the group home parents in the group certainly helped to kick-start this process.

BEYOND THE GROUP

Since the first group, a parent support/education group has run every year. It has been a continuous learning experience, and we have modified each group according to the specific needs of the parents and our own increased skill and experience level.

The length of the groups has increased from ten to twelve weeks. The extra two sessions has increased our flexibility to spend more time on topics the group needs or wants. For example, one of the most recent groups was particularly interested in the concept of self-esteem and requested a session focusing on how to build their own and their children's self-esteem. We developed a session on this topic and were able to give the parents what they needed without compromising the content of other group sessions.

We have also designed a pre- and post-test, directly linked to the topics covered and the goal and objectives of the group, to more formally evaluate the program. To date, this has yielded consistent results indicating positive change for parents in the group. We are now searching for a standardized instrument that could be used for evaluation purposes, as this would lend even further credibility to the results.

Over the past year, we trained two of the organization's youth care workers to facilitate the parent group and added an extra group per year to meet the increased demand. The group has attracted the attention of other agencies in the community, including the Foster Parents Association, and plans are underway to work in collaboration with this association to include the natural families with whom they work in the parent group. We were also recently asked by a supervisor with the Department of Health and Community Services to provide training and support to staff of other group homes in the province so that they could start their own parent groups.

A SPRINGBOARD FOR FAMILY INVOLVEMENT

Our ulterior motive in developing the parent group was to use this as an introduction to family involvement within the organization. In this regard, it was a huge success. The group sparked an interest in and awareness of parents that had not been there previously, and we were able to build on this to move family work forward in other areas.

Concurrent to the development of the parent group was the introduction of family involvement in the organization's group home program. Months of informal preparation went into this, with staff discussing on how and why we wanted to involve families and where to start. Training was provided to staff on involving families in residential programs and working with families. What appeared to be the easiest way to begin this process was to just bring parents into the home. We started with the parents who participated in our first group and expanded from there.

Parents began spending time at the home "hanging out," participating in social and recreational activities, assisting us with household and maintenance tasks, and lending us their expertise in specific areas. Our focus was on building relationships, tapping into parents' strengths, sending them the message that their involvement was critical to their child's treatment and that they were important, and using all of this to optimize the relationships between the parents and their children.

In one example, a mother who was a great cook prepared supper at the group home every Sunday. She arrived early in the morning, often armed with board games, and spent the day interacting with her son and the other young people in the program, including cooking supper (in which she often involved the young people). Young people and staff all looked forward to her arrival. The young people enjoyed her attention and the staff appreciated her assistance. Her son was proud of his mom's contribution to the program. It did not hurt that people raved about her cooking for days.

This mother also spent time in the unit on other occasions and participated in many activities with the young people and staff. Staff built strong relationships with her and she was quite open to feedback on her relationship with her son and things she could to ensure success when he returned home. The mom learned that she had a lot to offer and, instead of feeling like a failure because her son was in care, she used the placement as an opportunity to grow.

In another case, we had a father who was skilled at carpentry. In an effort to increase the level of interaction between him and his son and to help improve his own sense of self-worth and competency, we asked him to teach industrial arts once a week to the young people who were being home schooled at the group home. This provided a wonderful opportunity for the dad to make a positive contribution to the program, for the young people to learn new skills, and for the son to see his dad as someone others could look up to. While the dad was spending regular time at the group home, he noticed that we needed a new garbage box and shed and offered to make these for us. This turned into a summer long project that involved all of the young people.

Another parent, Jane, shared her talent for making crafts by teaching the young people to make Christmas decorations. While doing so, she demonstrated great patience and teaching skills, which staff pointed out to her. During one craft session, one of the young people refused to participate and arranged to be out of the house during the session. This young person had been involved in an altercation with Jane's son earlier in the week that had been initiated by Jane's son, and he appeared to think that Jane would have the same hostile feelings towards him that her son had. Jane picked up on this and waited in the unit for this young person to come home so she could give him an individual craft session. The young person appeared overwhelmed by her actions and beamed the whole time he was making his Christmas mailbox. Jane's son learned that his mom had her own opinions and could stand up to him (he had told her not to help this other young person). The benefits of her actions far exceeded anything staff could have done in this situation.

This same parent, along with her husband and daughter, were regular visitors to the group home. They often showed up on special occasions. In one case, a young person had reached a milestone in the group home program, and there was to be a party to celebrate. The parents of this young person were unable to attend, for various reasons. When Jane's son mentioned this to her, she and her family showed up during the celebration with a cake and a present for the young person. This made an ordinary celebration extraordinary for this young person.

Christmas parties have proven to be a surefire way to get families into the program; even the most reluctant parents will attend a Christmas party! The following story was relayed to me by the coordinator of the organization's two-bed intensive treatment program:

> A Christmas dinner was planned for December 20th and invitations were extended from Donny to his mother and from Tom to his mother and two teenage sisters, along with his father who he had not lived with for many years. Also included in the party were the program staff and the social worker. To add to everyone's list of things to do, a request was made for each person to provide one handmade gift that had something to say about the person receiving it.

The full Christmas meal for fourteen people was served around a single table, put together by adding a meeting table and a card table to the small kitchen set. Some around the table had never met. At the start of the meal, Tom's parents made several unkind remarks towards each other but the frequency diminished over the course of the meal. As the meal moved to dessert, everyone appeared relaxed and to be enjoying the company. There was even a hint of romance in the air between Tom's father and Donny's mother (which staff definitely did not encourage!).

When it was time to take turns presenting gifts, everyone was moved by the expressions of love and encouragement that were offered by family members. Tom's mother and sisters wrote poems to share the pride that, for the first time in his life, Tom was dealing with his issues in a positive way. Donny gave his mother a hand-made card that expressed his delight at getting to go home for Christmas (the previous year Donny had been remanded in custody during the season). The sentimentality was contagious at that point. The staff exchanged gifts of homemade cake, small artwork, and a crafted microphone that was later used for a few solo Christmas carols.

Quite unexpectedly, a Tuesday that started out with school and a busy day of work turned into a Christmas memory shared by an unlikely group of people.

There are many of these examples, and they are the reason that staff are committed to family involvement. Although the workload increased, so did the benefits. All of the homes within the organization have now moved in this direction. Program goals and objectives have been revised to highlight the importance of involving families, and the organization's mission statement has been adjusted accordingly. The strategic plan for the organization includes increasing the level and scope of family involvement in all programs. Staff embraced this concept, and all new staff are informed that working with families will be a part of their job.

REFERENCES

Anglin, J., & Glossop, R. (1993). Parent education and support: an emerging field for child and youth care work. In R. Ferguson, A. Pence, & C. Denholm (Eds.), *Professional child and youth care* (2nd ed.). Vancouver, BC: University of British Columbia Press.

Anglin, J. P. (1985). Developing education and support groups for parents of children in residential care. *Residential Group Care and Treatment, 3*(2), 15-27.

Bavelok, S. J. (1998). *Nurturing program for parents and adolescents.* Park City, Utah: Family Development Resources, Inc.

Child Welfare League of America (1992). *Newfoundland and Labrador Department of Social Services Child Protection Services Evaluation.* Unpublished document.

Garbarino, J. (1983). Social support networks: rx for the helping professions. In J. K. Whittaker, J. Garbarino, & Associates (Eds.), *Social support networks: informal helping in the human services.* New York: Aldine Publishing Company.

Garfat, T. (1990). The involvement of family members as consumers in treatment programs for troubled youths. In M. Krueger, & N. Powell (Eds.), *Choices in caring.* Washington, DC: Child Welfare League of America.

Garfat, T., & McElwee, C. N. (1991). The changing role of family in child and youth care practice. *Journal of Child and Youth Care Work, 15-16,* 236-248.

Garland, D. S. (1987). Residential child care workers as primary agents of family intervention. *Child and Youth Care Quarterly, 16*(1), 21-34.

Government of Newfoundland and Labrador (1997). *Executive summary: report of the review of the Child Welfare Act and program with proposals for future directions.* Unpublished document.

Grealish, E. M., Hawkins, R. P., Meadowcroft, P., Weaver, P., Frost, S. S., & Lynch, P. (1989). A behavioral group procedure for parents of severely troubled and troubling youth in out-of-home care: alternative to conventional parent training. *Child and Youth Care Quarterly, 18,* 49-61.

Halonen, J., Rilling, C., & Jensen, C. (1995). *Parent learning profile*. Park City, UT: Family Development Resources, Inc.

Halonen, J., Rilling, C., & Jensen, C. (1995). *Guide book for parent learning profile*. Park City, UT: Family Development Resources, Inc.

Jenson, J. M., & Whittaker, J. K. (1987). Parental involvement in residential treatment. *Children and Youth Services Review, 9*, 81-100.

Littauer, C. (1980). Working with families of children in residential treatment. *Child Welfare, 59*(4), 225-234.

Littner, N. (1975). The importance of the natural parents to the child in placement. *Child Welfare, 44*(3), 175-181.

Noble, D. N., & Gibson, D. (1994). Family values in action: family connectedness for children in substitute care. *Child and Youth Care Forum, 23*(5), 315-328.

Palmer, S. (1995). *Maintaining family ties: inclusive practice in foster care*. Washington, DC: Child Welfare League of America.

Peterson, R. W., & Brown, R. (1982). The child care worker as treatment coordinator and parent trainer. *Child Care Quarterly, 11*(3), 188-203.

Select Committee on Children's Interests (1996). *Listening & acting: a plan for child, youth, and community empowerment*. St. John's, New Foundland: House of Assembly.

VanderVen, K., & Stuck, E. N. (1995). Preparing agencies and workers for family contract services. *Journal of Child and Youth Care, 10*(3), 13-26.

Webster, C. D., Somjen, L., Sloman, L., Bradley, S., Mooney, S. A., & Mack, J. E. (1979). The child care worker in the family: some case examples and implications for the design of family-centered programs. *Child Care Quarterly, 8*(1), 5-18.

Finding Identity in Family Work: Community Child Care-Workers in Ireland

Niall C. McElwee

SUMMARY. The family has always enjoyed an elevated status in Ireland, yet it was not until the mid-1990s that family-based intervention work really found expression in a new division of child and youth care: community child care-workers. This paper introduces readers to an area of child and youth care work in Ireland devoted to an ecological understanding of the child "at risk" and working with the child and the child's family outside of a residential or institutional setting. The paper includes a brief interview with a community child care-worker, observations from a master's student in social care who has also worked in community child care, and concludes by reviewing 12 key areas community child care-workers must address if their status is to be secured in the Irish child and youth care landscape. *[Article copies available for a fee from The Haworth Document Delivery Service: 1-800-HAWORTH. E-mail address: <docdelivery@haworthpress.com> Website: <http://www.HaworthPress.com> © 2003 by The Haworth Press, Inc. All rights reserved.]*

KEYWORDS. Youthwork with families, youth care work, social work with families, family-centered residential care, child and youth care, family services, family support, parent education, residential care work and families

Niall C. McElwee is affiliated with the Centre for Child and Youth Care Learning, Athlone Institute of Technology, Ireland.

[Haworth co-indexing entry note]: "Finding Identity in Family Work: Community Child Care-Workers in Ireland." McElwee, Niall C. Co-published simultaneously in *Child & Youth Services* (The Haworth Press, Inc.) Vol. 25, No. 1/2, 2003, pp. 191-210; and: *A Child and Youth Care Approach to Working with Families* (ed: Thom Garfat) The Haworth Press, Inc., 2003, pp. 191-210. Single or multiple copies of this article are available for a fee from The Haworth Document Delivery Service [1-800-HAWORTH, 9:00 a.m. - 5:00 p.m. (EST). E-mail address: docdelivery@haworthpress.com].

The importance of the family was enshrined in the Irish Constitution of 1937. Perhaps the single greatest change since then is the movement away from an insular and closed understanding of Catholicity to a more open and pluralist society. Despite this nominal protection, Ireland was without an explicit family policy. Family affairs were the responsibility at the government level of a number of Ministries until the creation of a Family Affairs Unit within the Department of Social, Community, and Family Affairs in 1997 (Richardson, 1998). In the thinking that informed the *Commission on the Family Report (1998)*, six principles were noted:

1. Recognition that the family unit is a fundamental unit providing stability and well-being in our society.
2. The unique and essential family function is that of caring and nurturing for all its members.
3. Continuity and stability are major requirements in family relationships.
4. An equality of well-being is recognised between individual family members.
5. Family membership confers rights, duties and responsibilities.
6. A diversity of family forms and relationships should be recognised. (p. 4)

The Irish family looks very different today than it did just a couple of decades ago. Women are marrying later in life, one in three children are born outside of the marital unit, divorce is now part of the landscape, more women work outside the family home, and increasing numbers of men are stay-at-home dads. For many reasons, a minority of families are unable to cope with the circumstances in which they find themselves.

The past two decades in Ireland were a time of unparalleled development in child protection and welfare. Indeed, Irish society has changed beyond recognition for many. One of my favorite contemporary Irish novelists is from Finglas in Dublin, a man called Dermot Bolger. In one of Bolger's most controversial novels, *The Journey Home* (1990), the central character describes Dublin of the 1980s without any romantic idealism:

> . . . I gazed from the window at tumbledown lane outside. The sleeping children had gone. A man with a cardboard box and a blanket jealously guarded their spot. Far below, Dublin was moving towards the violent crescendo of its Friday night, taking to the twentieth century like an aborigine to whiskey. Studded punks pissed openly on corners. Glue sniffers stumbled into each other, coats over their arms as they tried to pick pockets. Addicts stalked rich-looking tourists. Stolen cars zigzagged through the distant grey estates where pensioners prayed anxiously behind bolted doors, listening for the smash of glass. In the new disco bars

children were queuing, girls of fourteen shoving their way up for last drinks at the bar. (p. 35)

This quote depicts the Dublin often seen through the point of view of a child and youth care worker and show how families can easily come into contact with human services.[1]

Families may engage with child protection services such as day services, residential services, or community-based services. In the community, there is a relatively new type of worker: the community child-care worker. Because I feel strongly that we need to reach children and youth as early as possible in their "at risk" biographies, I consider the community child-care worker post to be essential.

PROTECTING CHILDREN AND YOUTH "AT RISK"

The Child Care Act (1991), Children First Guidelines (1999), the National Children's Strategy (2000), and the Children's Act (2001) have all assisted in moving the child and young person to center stage. The two professional Associations–the Irish Association of Care Workers and the Resident Managers' Association–and the academic Association–the Irish Association of Social Care Educators–have politicized the marginalized child and young person to a degree that it is now impossible to ignore child and youth care issues. As Ireland is divided into Health Board regions (soon to be amalgamated), each Board assumes responsibility for children and youth in its geographical catchment. A major legal instrument, the 1991 Child Care Act, places a legal obligation on every Health Board to promote the welfare of children in its area who are not receiving adequate care and attention or are "at risk." The Act was phased in from 1991 to 1996. Prevention, early intervention, and a philosophy of supporting children in their own families and communities permeates the Act. A child may be removed from the family *only* in exceptional circumstances.

The 1991 Child Care Act, Section 8(2), notes that the categories of children who are likely to be recipients of family support services of the Health Boards are:

- Children whose parents are dead or missing;
- Children whose parents have deserted or abandoned them;
- Children who are in care of the Health Board;
- Children who are homeless;
- Children who are at risk of being neglected or ill-treated; and
- Children whose parents are unable to care for them due to ill-health or for any other reason.

The Act provides for a Supervision Order, which is crucial for the community child care-worker as it offers an opportunity whereby a child may be protected in cases of suspected abuse without taking the traumatic step of removing the child from the family home. Section 3(1) of the Act provides that it shall be the function of every Health Board to promote the welfare of children in its area who are not receiving adequate care and attention. The Health Boards must be active in this process, and I have been critical of their failure to do so in the past, particularly in relation to juvenile involvement in prostitution (McElwee, 1998).

In all of this new thinking there is acceptance that it is poor practice to attempt to work with children and young people in isolation. A child must be reached in the context of being part of a family where he or she ultimately belongs and, in the main, would like to return. Interestingly, 33% of children in care in Ireland in the early 1990s were there not because they were delinquent, but because their parents simply could not cope (Gilligan, 1991).

Being a father of only some 18 months I have a fresh and new outlook on child protection and welfare. I have seen, first hand, the effects of sleep deprivation and role allocation of couples. It is difficult to cope with a screaming and demanding child when there are two loving and well-meaning parents at the best of times, but when there are a series of other serious stressors on the relationship, one can understand how quickly familial meltdown can occur. Madge's (1986) notion of an ABC of risk (age of parents, burdens carried by parents, consistency and change in the lives of children, dynamic of the family and experiences within the family) are clear markers for family riskness and should not be ignored.

THE COMMUNITY CHILD CARE-WORKER IN CONTEXT

Social Care is the term used in Ireland for the provision of care, protection, support, welfare, and advocacy for vulnerable or dependent clients—individually or in groups. This is achieved through the planning and evaluation of individualised and group programs of care that are based on needs, identified in consultation with the client, and delivered through day-to-day shared life experiences. All interventions are supposed to be based on established best practice and in-depth knowledge of life-span development.

It has taken some time, but a role matrix for the Irish social care practitioner has been identified under separate constellations with nine key task areas including "organiser, planner, team-member, attachment builder, leader, liaison person, programmer, counsellor and therapeutic teacher" (Graham, 2002). The core employment in child and youth care in Ireland resides in residential child care centres within the Education, Health and Justice system, but it was the publication of the *Task Force Report on Child Care Services* (1981) that signaled a shift from residential services to community and family. This report acknowledged that the family home is the most appropriate location for intervention. Thus, the concept of the community child care-worker was born, but it was not a birth without complications. As the 1998 IMPACT Report suggests, the rapid development of the position was not preceded by any policy document, planning, or forethought which, in turn, contributed to the role being allowed to develop in an ad hoc and haphazard way that depended often on the personality of the manager or child care-workers rather than any clear definition or guidelines (IMPACT, 1998).

Nonetheless, there is a stated emphasis on partnership, and this is to be welcomed. The IMPACT (1998) Report acknowledges that partnership is accomplished by:

1. Enabling children to return home where needs are best met.
2. Enabling children to return home from care and prevent reoccurrence of the difficulties which initially caused them to be placed in care by planning and preparing families for the move and working closely with them throughout.
3. Promote positive parenting, interactions and experiences between parents and children.
4. Developing and participating in group work.
5. Liaison with other professional agencies.
6. Supervision and observation, in particular with other professionals on the team preparing children for leaving care.
7. Co-work in child protection, in particular with other professionals on the team preparing children for leaving care.
8. Court work.
9. Community networking, i.e., schools, neighbourhood youth projects, community playgroups and youth clubs and detecting children at risk (p. 33).

In a national population of approximately 3.75 million people, there are only about 85 community child care-workers, and this is with an estimated 25% of our children and youth living in poverty! The community child care-worker is a trained, highly skilled worker who works with children in partnership with their families in the community. The key word here is *partnership*. Community child care-workers are responsible for individual work with children where a particular need is highlighted. They are required to engage in therapeutic and development programs with children and adolescents and are involved, at all levels, in prevention and intervention work. Their education and training equips them to work directly with children and adolescents providing therapeutic and developmental programs to children identified as having particular needs, such as the need for regular and planned intellectual stimulation, the need for assistance in changing problematic behavior, or the need for support in adjusting to significant family traumas.

The community child care-workers also provide encouragement and skills training to parents and to foster carers who are challenged by the demands of caring for children. They regularly arrange and assist with access visits between parents and their children in care. They help children who are planning to leave a care placement to prepare for their return home or for independent living (South Eastern Health Board, 1998, p. 27).

Approximately 95% of the 85 community child care-workers are female, 22% hold Degrees in Social Care, 49% hold Diplomas in Social Studies, 29% hold Diplomas in Child Care with only 34% being employed more than five years (Ryan, 2000). Put somewhat differently, the majority of community child-care workers are young, female, and have been employed for only a brief period when one compares the discipline to the more established residential child care provision. Community child care-workers are perceived as infants in the general Irish child care system and are attempting to position themselves as key players in working with vulnerable families.

One area of work that particularly emphasizes partnership is that of aftercare planning and development which might involve families of origin, alternative carers (foster carers or residential care staff) social workers, youth training workshops, supported lodgings, community welfare officers, and a range of other individuals and agencies. Aftercare plans are tailored to the needs of the individual young person (South Eastern Health Board, 1998). Much of the community child care-worker's role is around prevention work, which has its roots in the 1960s when it was suggested that concepts and frameworks derived from public health programs could also be applicable in the socioemotional fields. The concept did not broaden in Ireland until the 1980s when Holman (1988) suggested that a range of services be developed along a continuum ranging from clinical to neighborhood and community development type models. Indeed, one could argue that community child care did not come into its own until the passing of the 1991 Child Care Act and increased economic prosperity–the so-called Celtic tiger economy when the national unemployment fell below 3%. Of course, as with tigers in the wild, the Celtic version is now becoming extinct and this has had a knock-on effect on the willingness of the government to resource child care.

WORKING WITH VULNERABLE FAMILIES

The family is the single most important influence in a child's life. Recognition of this has influenced the way that most Western European and North

American child-care systems deal with the care and protection of vulnerable children and youth. Placement of children outside of the home is now more often viewed as a support to the family rather than as substitute care, and social care practitioners, whether working in a residential or community setting, have a key role to play in working with the child's family. There is always a danger that social care practitioners may alienate a family, particularly the parent or parents, out of a misguided sense of the welfare of a child, thinking that the family is necessarily the problem. Whilst this is sometimes the case, we must respect the fact that a child or young person will very often want to be with her family even if "expert" systems consider it to be entirely problematic. Child and youth care must attempt to work with the family to reach a child. Parents have, at least, some skills and these could be targeted to create a sense of ownership.

In an editorial for the *Journal of Child and Youth Care*, Thom Garfat (2001) rightly observes that the family is crucial. He notes the following in relation to working with children and youth:

- These are not our children.
- The residential facility is not home. Families are not the enemy.
- The more we divide the work, the more we divide the family.
- The residential centre is a support to family.
- Building on what you know is easier than starting over.
- It is easier to modify a program than to get funding for a new one.
- The more support that is available the easier it is for everyone.
- There is a cultural demand for residential programs to change in this way (Garfat, 2001).

Entering into the residential child-care system is always difficult. In discussing a pilot program in South Africa for children in residential care, Gaffley (2000) notes that temporary placements can become indeterminate sentences with "drifters" in the system and loss of family contact. Gaffley is concerned that many children will know no one outside the safety of the residential unit, leaving both the young person and the family of origin with deep emotional scarring. Thus there is a moral and ethical responsibility to achieve clarity and consistency in our human services provision. Triseliotis (1983), for example, acknowledges that young people require knowledge about their backgrounds, which is important for identity formation and emotional adjustment. An important role, then, for the community child-care worker is to assist the young person in obtaining and retaining this knowledge.

Family Support

Family support services were developed largely as a cross between a home visitation model and an intensive family preservation strategy aimed to target high-risk families (O'Reilly, 2002). It is worth mentioning that the experience of family support in the United States of America is not radically different. Whittaker (1993) argues that family support "reflects more a set of values than a clearly defined program strategy" (p. 6).

In the Irish context, Gilligan (1995) has identified six key principles for family support:

1. Low-key, nonclinical and user friendly in approach.
2. Operates on the principle of consent rather than coercion.
3. Aim to enhance rather than diminish the confidence of those helped.
4. Needs a purposeful focused quality mostly, but "being there" may be important sometimes.
5. In "protective" mode, it should focus on a particular targeted problem, for a specific time-period, and with specific and measurable outcomes.
6. Geared to what works best in a particular set of circumstances (p. 71).

RELATIONSHIP CONSTRUCTION IN CHILD AND YOUTH CARE

My experience suggests that the vast majority of community child care-workers accept the concept that child and youth care is based on a belief in the power of relationship in influencing human growth and development (Brendtro, 1969; Trieschman, 1969). The translation of this belief into effective practice requires a definition of relationship as an organic process and an understanding of the range of relationships that may occur. Relationships are the essence of child and youth care practice, for it is within the context of meaningful relationships that young people may frame their experiences. The attention to relationship and being-in-relationship while utilizing everyday life events for therapeutic purposes is one of the ways in which the professional practice of child and youth care work distinguishes itself from other forms of helping and caring (Garfat, 2001).

Garfat (2001a) gave a lovely example of this in his keynote speech in Drogheda, Ireland, when he recounted for us an experience he had with a youth in residential care. Thom and the teen were both shaving in front of a mirror one morning, and Thom used the opportunity to enter into a discussion on life with the chap who had proven difficult to reach. Thom used their mutual shaving experience as a therapeutic moment captured. As much of the work of a community child care-worker is done in the house of origin or an aftercare unit, there are many such possibilities if the worker is attuned to relationship.

Ricks (CYC-Net, 2001) suggests that child and youth care practice does not occur within a vacuum but within the relationship that develops between the practitioner and the client(s). It occurs in light of the multiple relationships that the practitioner and the client(s) have with the rest of the world. The process of practice involves the practitioner, the client(s), their families, the official ministries that are involved, the community, the organizations of all parties, ad infinitum. It is this web of relationships that creates and adds to the complexity of the practice process and as child and youth care practitioners we are in the middle of it.

There is no doubt that community child care-workers are highly valued by the children and youth with whom they work. In the most recent study completed in this area, Kane (2002) found that 90% of the sample group felt "that they were always listened to" by the community child care-worker. When asked how they would rate their relationship with the community child care-worker on a scale of 1 to 10 (1 is poor and 10 is excellent), 100% of the respondents rated between 8 and 10. Again, 100% of the respondents stated that they could be honest regarding things that were important or troubling them. Kane says that "the recurring theme from respondents is that the relationship they have with the community child care-worker is one of trust, honesty and support" (p. 81).

Perhaps more than any other discipline of Irish child and youth care, the community child care-worker has an opportunity to develop a sustained relationship over time as the community child care-worker is enabled, by virtue of the post, to stay with a child or young person over a period of time in the child's or young person's space.

I might now include some brief commentary from Susan, a community child care-worker, to illustrate this point.[2]

TALES FROM THE COALFACE:
ON BEING A COMMUNITY CHILD CARE-WORKER

Susan is 30 and holds a national diploma and degree in Social Care, and most recently she worked for a Health Board in the south of Ireland. She worked in community child-care for a period of some 19 months (after working in day care and consultancy) prior to taking maternity leave. Susan worked in a multidisciplinary team in a community care facility on a team including some 12 social workers, two permanent community child care-workers and four clinical psychologists. She had a case-load of 21 clients.

N: How did you come to be involved in community child care?

S: By accident. I had been working in day care and had taken a break to renovate an old cottage. I was interested in another area of child and youth care and one day received a call from a social worker based in a particular Health Board area. The Board wanted a child and youth care worker to engage in direct work with a particular family, and from this I was offered part-time work which eventually panned out into full-time work as a community child care-worker.

N: What did you like most about the job?

S: Building up relationships with people and especially the children. Being able to implement programs with children and, crucially, being able to see these programs making a difference in their lives. I liked travelling to different areas and the fact that when I went into work on any given day, I could end up doing a multitude of tasks such as family work, life-story work, and the like.

N: What did you like least about the job?

S: The reporting structure. Not being seen by our peers as professionals in our own right. Not having our own full team of community child care-workers and not been given the same footing as the other related professions such as social work.

N: What are your key concerns in relation to community child care?

S: There are a number of different things from a professional point of view. The new pay scales, for example, may mean that the Health Board will not employ many community child care-workers with a small minority of professionals. It will be difficult to move up the pay scales as we won't have people to fight for our cause for team leader positions and the like. There is also a strong crossover between social workers, family support workers and community child care-workers confusing the work terrain for all of us with no clarity between us. From a work practice point of view, it is dangerous driving around violent clients.

N: Can you describe for me a typical client, if such a person exists?

S: He doesn't exist because I covered the spectrum of life from early years to older adults. Primarily, the children with whom I worked were either in foster care, supported lodgings, or residential care.

N: Can you describe for me a typical working day in community child care?

S: I arrived into work at about 9.00 a.m. and looked up my diary to see what was booked in from earlier weeks. Work could involve, for example, my first session with a parenting program with parents, followed by collecting children on an access visit having traveled twenty miles to pick them up. After lunch I might engage in supporting a child in care, maybe use of self-esteem programs, a supervised access, aftercare program with a child who was about to leave care.

The variety of work cited by Susan is not uncommon to community child careworkers in any of the geographical areas around Ireland.

THE KEY ISSUES IN MOVING FORWARD THE AGENDA OF COMMUNITY CHILD CARE

I want to examine 12 key issues that affect community child care-workers as they practice with youth and their families in Ireland today. Of course, this list is only intended to open up the debate and does not claim to be definitive. I am sure that the community child care-workers could well add several additional issues.

Finding an Identity

Perhaps the first concern is around the discipline finding its own identity. Is child and youth care, for example, a discipline or a profession? This discipline/ profession argument has been well debated in the past with Merriam-Webster, (1995) stating that a profession refers to "a calling requiring specialised knowledge and often long academic preparation." Gaughan and Gharabaghi (1999) argue that a discipline becomes professional when engaging in it requires prior skills and knowledge distinct from the skills and knowledge one would require to engage in other disciplines.

It seems to me that community child care-workers are stuck in no-person's land somewhere in the middle between being perceived as "mini-social workers," on the one hand, and as evolving child-care practitioners on the other. This actually applies to all child and youth care practice in Ireland with various statutory and non-statutory groups attempting to clarify that the work of child careworkers is distinguishable from other professions (Department of Health and Children, 2000a, 2000b):

* By duration and intensity of the relationships with the client.
* The range of ages and the variety of needs of the clients within such a long-term context.
* The extension of this work into the family and community.

Surprisingly, one of O' Reilly's (2002) community child care-workers was unclear of what the job would entail, despite the fact that she had spent three years in college studying social care. She stated, *"I knew it was based in the community, but other than that I wasn't sure . . . I was very unclear then"* (p. 30). This lack of clarity may be attributed to the college training programs where, perhaps, inadequate attention is given to structured classes on the different areas of child and youth care such as community work. Students have often complained to me that academic programs overly concentrate on residential child care theory (at the expense of project and community work) but, conversely, resident managers have informed me that colleges do not emphasise residential care to the extent that they would like and that a majority of our graduates have to be either retrained or reoriented. What is one to do?

There is no denying that community child care-workers have not formally published widely in their field detailing for students or instructors, what it is they *do* on a daily basis. There are, for example, no papers from community child care-workers in either the peer-reviewed *Irish Journal of Applied Social Studies* or the Irish *Journal of Child Centred Practice*, so one is forced to rely on anecdotal evidence or attempt to patch together a portfolio from a range of publications that deal briefly or in passing with the post, such as the Health Board Annual Reviews or student dissertations.[3] In its annual review of child care and family support services the South Eastern Health Board notes that the daily work completed across four geographical areas is quite diverse, with Waterford concentrating more on the seven areas of service provision than the other three areas. This may partly be explained by numbers of service users, but is also about the identity held by staff across these areas (South Eastern Health Board, 1998).

A Distinct Philosophy

A second issue is around locating and agreeing on a *distinct* philosophy and worldview. It seems to me that community child care-work in Ireland has not actually developed and articulated an indigenous philosophy or worldview; that is to say, the philosophy of community child care-workers work is still evolving, emergent, or emerging. It is really a hodge-podge of theory and practice from a number of divergent professions and philosophies. This is, of course, part of a wider phenomenon in child and youth care where change and uncertainty pervade the work environment. An example provided by one of my social care master's degree candidates, Fiona Clarke, from her field practicum experience is that social workers were often quite unclear about the specific role(s) of community child care-workers when attempting to supervise them, resulting in supervision sessions that did not maximize potential for either party (Fiona Clarke, personal communication, March 6, 2003). Until there is agreement around a philosophy of practice, it will be difficult to mobilize as a political unit to effect greater services for at-risk families and status for the community child care-workers.

Developing Professional Status

A third issue is around maintaining and developing the aforementioned *professional* status. This most certainly is one of the key areas for community child care-workers in that they consistently claim to be professional but are unable to articulate many of the particular traits associated with the more established professions.[4] Of course, this debate has been going on in North America since the late 1950s, but it is relatively new here in Ireland (McElwee, 1998; Stuart, 1998, 2000).

Examples of this new interest abound. The word "profession" appears again and again in various in-house publications (Gilligan, 1991; IMPACT, 1998; Ryan, 2000).

I want to briefly identify four issues with claiming professional status; the first is that in using the term "profession" it assumes that one has achieved autonomy. Second, it assumes that one wants to achieve recognition from peers. Third, it assumes that there is respect for one's work. Fourth, it assumes that the boundaries of community child care-work have been developed. Unfortunately, to varying degrees, none of those four criteria have been adequately addressed. Child and youth care, as is practiced in Ireland today, could not be considered an autonomous profession, as is argued the case with nursing which has experienced many similar struggles. Indeed, one could argue about whether or not child and youth care should want to be considered an autonomous profession. Recently, Stewart (2001), discussing North America, has argued that child and youth care should be seen more as a craft than as a profession. In a craft each product is a little different and the work cannot be standardized since it depends on the uniqueness of the parts and how they come together for the whole.

There are a series of theoretical approaches to viewing professionalism. Berube (1984) and Kelly (1990) adopt a functionalist approach to professionalism by addressing service to people, formal education, and an organised and distinct body of knowledge, clientele, and colleagues that recognise your authority, code of ethics, professional culture, professional association, autonomy, and self-regulation. If we look at this in the Irish context we can see that there are a number of these missing. Again, for example, there is no established code of ethics agreed upon by all the actors in child and youth care. The organised and distinct body of knowledge is, in the main, not indigenous to Ireland as we have drawn extensively from European and United Kingdom-based social work and clinical psychology practice, which I have critiqued in the past.

Perhaps surprisingly, it is only recently that we have looked extensively to North America for literature on child and youth care. I have traveled to all of the Irish third-level colleges presenting papers on child and youth care identity in the recent past and, many times, I have been astounded to hear that degree (and post-degree) students have not heard of what I would consider to be key North American authors such as Fritz Redl, Albert Trieschman, James Whittaker, Larry Brendtro, Henry Maier, Penny Parry or Karen VanderVen to name but some of the established commentators. The CYC-Net is still largely unheard of in many college sites. Added to this, it is almost as if we are afraid to listen to our own emerging voices for fear that they are not valid and this has held back the advancement of child and youth care in this country.

Running for the Border

A fourth issue is around establishing and sustaining a *definitive* qualification border around hard-won "achieved" status. At least one health board area employs individuals as community child care-workers without the necessary National Diploma in Applied Social Studies Social Care or BA in Social Care. Clarke (personal communication, March 6, 2003) comments that in her field practicum, there was a feeling amongst the community child care-workers that a diploma sufficed for the post, despite the articulated national agenda of Degree.

It is the responsibility of the community child care-worker community itself to establish and sustain borders around their achieved status, as employers will always minimize resource spending where possible and opt for those "training but not fully trained." Of course, this is easier said than done when the group itself is so fragmented and dispersed throughout the country.

Nonetheless, a start must be made. Perhaps the strength here is that, as a discipline, community child care has the highest concentration of diploma and degree holders per capita in social care. To their credit, community child care-workers established a subgroup within the representative professional body, the Irish Association of Care Workers, and have organized their own subconferences as with the one held in Portlaoise in 2001, and these must be seen as positive developments and an effort to politicise themselves.

Entry and Exit Wounds

A fifth issue is agreeing upon the points of entry into and exit from community child care-work. Again, it is a responsibility of the community child care-workers to get their respective health board managers to agree on points of entry into and exit from community child care-work, to have these set down in writing, and to have these as part of formal contracts.

In my interview with her, Fiona Clarke (personal communication, March 6, 2003) stated that, "Meetings would often break down because the team would argue over what exactly was required for permanency and administration was deliberately vague and unclear. Ill-feeling, then, pervaded the team's sense of ownership around community child care."

One might argue, for example, that only holders of social care or child and youth care degrees could work as a *professional* community child care-worker. This might create a positive status around the posts that has more to do with a sense of identity than merely wanting not to work in residential child care. It would certainly make the situation clearer for students and graduates with an interest in this particular area of work.

Promoting Expertise

A sixth issue is that of agreeing on areas of community child-care expertise that mark this work out from the expertise and experiences of colleagues in related but different areas. Again, from reading through transcripts of interview data and from some of the limited emerging documentation, one could argue that relationship is perhaps the key area of expertise community child care-workers have in terms of working with the entire family as opposed to a single child (Ryan, 2000). Although we are talking about relatively new positions, community child care-workers tend to stay in employment in the same location over periods of time, which allows for the genuine cultivation of relationships. It is not uncommon for the turnover rate in residential care to be some 30% of staff in any given twelve-month period in some centers, and this is simply not the case with the community child-care network.

Encroachment

A seventh issue is what to do about family-support workers and the increasing allocation to them by health board managers of roles seen by many established direct workers to be the preserve of community child care-workers. This is a highly political area to stray into. Nonetheless, anecdotal evidence suggests that family-support workers often get travel expenses from their home base rather than a central base, and this has annoyed many community child care-workers as this is not the case with their posts. Also, the qualification base of the family-support workers is typically (but not always) significantly lower than the community child care-worker.

Certainly, it makes economic sense for the health boards to go down the road of employing more and more family-support workers as they are less expensive to employ than the community child care-workers as we operate in an increasingly resource depleted world. The moves to formally train family-support workers is being watched with interest by the Irish Association of Social Care Educators.

On Being Separated from a Wider Team

An eighth issue is, as our friends in real estate would say, location, location, location. Community child care-workers are often based in satellite health centers for part of their day where there is little contact with the rest of the multidisciplinary team for full-day periods. Both Susan's and Fiona's experience was that older clients tended to be visited in their homes or a neutral location such as a coffee shop, but younger clients tended to come into the health center to a dedicated family room. This room was shared by social workers and community child care-workers.

Feeling part of a team is very significant in establishing an identity. One of the challenges facing community child care-workers is the historical emphasis on residential child-care provision with team identity located in one building, or more recently a group of small homes. Thus, one identified with "St. Hilda's Unit" or "St. Gerard's Home" (not their real names) and the staff therein. This is not the case with the community child care-workers who continually state that they feel "on their own."

The fact that they are asked to work for extended periods of times by themselves with volatile clients is potentially dangerous. Susan, for example, worked at least 1 day in every 10 some fourteen miles from base for periods of between 1 and 2 hours with individual clients and their families, often with no other community child care-worker present.

Finding a Team

A ninth difficulty is being part of a social work/psychology team as opposed to a community child care-worker team. Again, this is part of the undeveloped philosophy and agenda of community child care-workers, but community child care-workers often end up as an appendage to a social work or clinical psychologist team with, perhaps, only one colleague for moral support. One might consider it to be good practice that community child care-workers would have their own reporting teams with their own reporting structures. Clarke recounts that during her practicum in community child care, weekly team meetings were often unattended by social workers, but community child care-workers were present approximately 90% of the time. This led to serious levels of dissatisfaction from both groups of workers (personal communication, March 6, 2003).

Doing the Work of Others

A tenth issue facing community child care is that of being asked to undertake programs that one has little formal training for, or is considered to be the work of another discipline. Again, anecdotal evidence suggests that community child care-workers are frequently given unwanted work tasks by (their senior) social work colleagues; tasks that are not viewed by community child care-workers as being their roles. An example of such a role is securing accommodation for a client on a Friday evening when the social work team has gone home which Susan had to do on several occasions. There are, of course, potentially disastrous legal implications if something goes wrong. Again and again we see that a central difficulty is that community child care-workers' roles are not adequately defined in writing thus leaving their post open to abuse.

Freedom of Information

An eleventh issue lies in the Data Protection Act 1988, which allows clients to access material held on file about them. This has obvious implications for recording such as how to write up information around allegations of abuse, and very specific training is required in this area. This training is often given whilst on the job, and one is at the mercy of departmental budgets on this one. Much funding is given over to child sexual abuse programs and report writing falls low on the to-do list.

Managers Facilitating Development

Finally, there is a very strong perceived reluctance from management to facilitate community child care-workers attending meetings and training that is set up specifically for them by peers or colleagues in related areas–such as in the colleges. I have heard it articulated from around the country, and within different health board regions, that there is a stated reluctance from management to facilitate community child care-workers attending regional meetings and training as "priority is often placed elsewhere," the implication being that social workers find it easier to secure blocked time for training. It is, again, the responsibility of community child care-workers to become involved in planning their own training and self-development if they want to develop specialties.

CONCLUSION

Back in 1999 Thom Garfat observed that, "We put workers with typically a limited education in direct child and youth care practice . . . together with some of the most damaged, hurt and troubled youth of our society and expect them to be therapeutic, to help youth and families heal–to work minor miracles" (p. iii). Thankfully, the community child care-worker is typically trained to a nationally acceptable standard.

All of my above comments should be seen in the light of the idea that what is good for the community child care-worker is ultimately good for the child and young person with whom she works. Simply put, the community child care-worker is good for the family and is a post that deserves our full support–as does the family. I recently asked a residential child care-worker what he liked best about his work, and his answer was "going home." The fact that this care practitioner is only 25 and newly qualified perplexes me greatly. I worry about the long-term motivation of our young graduates.

Despite the twelve issues I have raised, community child care-work remains consistently as number one choice of destination amongst third-level students I have surveyed across all the Higher Education and Training Awards Accredited college sites in Ireland. I have lost count of the number of requests I have received from residential child care staff asking me to try and locate employment for them in the community.

Community child care-workers must be more proactive in contributing to the formal discourse at a social, policy, practice, and academic level. They could, for instance, publish in the *Irish Journal of Applied Social Studies*, a dedicated journal that is peer reviewed and is both practice and academic led. It is very supportive to hear the views of people in practice. Community child care-workers need to organize into a coherent representative voice. They must be prepared to politicize themselves and their roles, for it is in this landscape that advocacy takes place. A community child care-worker herself, Kane (2002) suggests, "Community Child Care intervention may be seen as a pathway in providing the unified vision of an Ireland where young people are respected and valued as young citizens" (p. 87). I heartily agree.

NOTES

1. I sometimes feel that my mental map of Ireland is contexted not in geographical lines or streets, but in child and youth care centres, drop-in centres, homeless shelters, and youth prisons, for I have come to know intimately where each of these is located in the towns and cities of this country. In each of these reside children and young people who have at least one thing in common: All have families.

2. I should declare my loyalties and note that Susan is my wife!
3. There are, however, a number of student dissertations in this area. These remain on file in the respective college library sites.
4. I have argued in the past that an obsession with achieving professional status is the Holy Grail for Irish child and youth care (see McElwee, 1998).

REFERENCES

Berube, P. (1984). Professionalisation of child care. A Canadian example. *Journal of Child Care, 2*(1), 13-26.
Bolger, D. (1990). *The journey home.* London: Penguin.
Brendtro, L. K. (1969). Establishing relationships beachheads. In A. E. Trieschman, J. K. Whittaker, & L. K. Brendtro (Eds.), *The other 23 hours.* Chicago: Aldine.
Child Care Act. (1991). Dublin: Government Publications.
Children's Act. (2001). Dublin: Government Publications.
Commission on the Family. (1998). *Strengthening families for life: Final report to the Minister for Social, Community and Family Affairs.* Dublin: Commission on the Family.
Department of Health and Children. (2000a). *Role of professional bodies and registration structures in the context of a statutory registration system.* Dublin: DOHC.
Department of Health and Children. (2000b). *Workshop on statutory registration for health and social care professionals.* Dublin: DOHC.
Gaffley, M. (2000, June). Work with families. *CYC On-Line, No. 17.*
Garfat, T. (1998). The effective child and youth care practitioner: A phenomenological inquiry. *Journal of Child and Youth Care, 12,* 1-2.
Garfat, T. (1999). Editorial: On reading about the child and youth care approach, *Journal of Child and Youth Care, 13*(1), iii-vii.
Garfat, T. (2001). Editorial. Congruence between supervision and practice. *Journal of Child and Youth Care, 15*(2), 111-1V.
Gaughan, P., & Gharabaghi, K. (1999). The prospects and dilemmas of child and youth care work as a professional discipline. *Journal of Child and Youth Care, 13*(1), 1-18.
Gilligan, R. (1991). *Irish child care services: Policy, practice and provision.* Dublin: Institute of Public Administration.
Graham, G. (2002). *A role matrix for the Irish social care worker.* Paper to the 2nd Annual Conference of the Irish Association of Social Care Educators. Carlow, Ireland.
Holman, B. (1988). *Putting families first.* London: MacMillan.
IMPACT. (1998). *Submission to the expert review group on behalf of care workers.* Dublin: Author.
IMPACT. (2000). *Final report of the expert group on the various health professions.* Dublin: Author.
Irish Social Policy Association. (1998). *Papers from panel discussion on the report of the Commission on the Family.* Dublin: Author.
Kane, N. (2002). *Community child care intervention. the foster child's experience.* Unpublished dissertation. Athlone: Athlone Institute of Technology.
Kelly, C. (1990). Professionalising child and youth care: An overview. In J. Anglin, C. Denholm, & A. Pence (Eds.), *Perspectives in professional child and youth care* (pp. 167-176). New York: The Haworth Press, Inc.

Madge, N. (Ed.). (1983). *Families at risk.* London: Heinmann.

McElwee, C. N. (1998). Juvenile prostitution: Ethical issues. In *Child prostitution in Ireland.* Dublin: Focus Ireland.

McElwee, C. N. (1998a). The search for the Holy Grail in Ireland: Social care in perspective. *Irish Journal of Applied Social Studies, 1*(1), 79-107.

National Children's Strategy. (2000). Dublin: Department of Health and Children.

O' Reilly, R. (2002). *The family support worker and the community child care worker: What is their role?* Unpublished doctoral dissertation. Athlone: Athlone Institute of Technology.

Pringle, M. (1986). *The needs of children.* London: Routledge.

Richardson, V. (1998). Foreword. *Papers from panel discussion on the Report of the Commission on the Family.* Dublin: ASPA.

Ryan, M. (2000). Unpublished dissertation. Athlone: Athlone Institute of Technology.

South Eastern Health Board. (1998). *Annual review of child care services 1997.* Kilkenny: Author.

Stuart, C. (1998, February 5). *Response to McElwee: A profession.* CYC-Net.

Stuart, C. (2000, June 3). *Response to McElwee: Certification.* CYC-Net.

Stewart, C. (2001). Professionalising child and youth care: Continuing the Canadian journey. *Journal of Child and Youth Care Work,* 15-16, 264-282.

Trieschman, A. E. (1969). Understanding the nature of a therapeutic milieu. In A. E. Trieschman, J. K. Whittaker, & L. K. Brendtro (Eds.), *The other 23 hours.* Chicago: Aldine de Gruyter.

Triseliotis, J. (1983). Identity and security in adoption and long-term foster care, *Adoption and Fostering, 77*(1), 22-31.

Whittaker, J. (1993). Changing paradigms in child and family services: Challenges for practice, policy and research. In H. Ferguson, R. Gilligan, & R. Torode (Eds.), *Surviving childhood adversity.* Dublin: Trinity Social Studies Press.

Moving to Youth Care Family Work in Residential Programs: A Supervisor's Perspective on Making the Transition

Mark Hill

Thom Garfat

SUMMARY. As work with families has become more popular in residential work with troubled youth, more and more programs are attempting to make the transition to being family-focused. There is much to be considered before starting this work. In this writing, a number of issues are highlighted which, from a supervisor's perspective, are essential to making a successful transition. This writing draws on the work done by the Nexus team in making the transition from an individual to a family-focused residential program. *[Article copies available for a fee from The Haworth Document Delivery Service: 1-800-HAWORTH. E-mail address: <docdelivery@haworthpress.com> Website: <http://www.HaworthPress.com> © 2003 by The Haworth Press, Inc. All rights reserved.]*

KEYWORDS. Youthwork with families, youth care work, social work with families, family-centered residential care, child and youth care, family services, family support, parent education, residential care work and families

---

Mark Hill is affiliated with Nexus, Nova Scotia. Thom Garfat is affiliated with TransformAction Consulting & Training, Montreal, Quebec, and is Co-editor of *CYC-Net* (www.cyc-net.org) and *Relational Child and Youth Care Practice*.

[Haworth co-indexing entry note]: "Moving to Youth Care Family Work in Residential Programs: A Supervisor's Perspective on Making the Transition." Hill, Mark, and Thom Garfat. Co-published simultaneously in *Child & Youth Services* (The Haworth Press, Inc.) Vol. 25, No. 1/2, 2003, pp. 211-223; and: *A Child and Youth Care Approach to Working with Families* (ed: Thom Garfat) The Haworth Press, Inc., 2003, pp. 211-223. Single or multiple copies of this article are available for a fee from The Haworth Document Delivery Service [1-800-HAWORTH, 9:00 a.m. - 5:00 p.m. (EST). E-mail address: docdelivery@haworthpress.com].

Digital Object Identifier: 10.1300/J024v25n01_13

Some assume that all programs and all youth care workers should be doing family work. This assumption may not fit all programs and could cause problems for both programs and individual workers if family work is started without first assessing the strengths, weaknesses, and purpose of the proposed program. Not all programs are prepared or designed to delve immediately into work with families. In the following we explore and focus primarily on the beginnings of family work within one program: the hurdles, the challenges, and the things we learned along the way. The perspective is that of a supervisor and highlights all that went well and the many things that went wrong.

> The first thing a team must decide prior to working with families, is why they want to do so. Yes, of course it is wonderful, exciting, and challenging and, of course, working with families will help your work with youth, maybe . . .

ABOUT BELIEFS

One essential belief in work with families is that "all youth have family" whether the family is immediate, extended, or found. Blood may not always be the basis for determining family.

In the residential programs where we have worked and in other programs with which we have had contact, communication with parents was often limited to:

- So, how was Alan's weekend? Or,
- Yes, I know Alan can react when you tell him "no." Or,
- Of course you can bring him home early from his home visit.

Let's begin with these statements.

One must believe that youth belong with family, yet it has been common in many programs that youth might go home to visit only on the weekends. This used to be the case in many programs. The truth is, a philosophy of visiting home on the weekends is one of the biggest hindrances to effective family work. You do not "visit" home. Going home and being at home is not a privilege one should have to earn. It must be seen as a right and one that is essential to any program working with youth and families. In residential care we may do brilliant life-skills training, awesome art classes, exceptional group meetings, great school programs, and many other in-facility programs. All of these programs typically occur within the residential facility, however, and if all the work is done there, you are not entering the family's world.

Once you begin the transition to working with families you begin to see that it is the family home, the living room, the kitchen, the front lawn, the lobby of the apartment building, and the garage that is the center of a family's world. This is where the stress, the hurt, and the love reside. It is where some of the best family work takes place. There is a tendency for people to want to be together only when things are going well.

We believe it is important that families learn how to be together in both good and bad times. Bringing a child back to the residential facility just because things are not going well in most cases only leads to feelings of failure for both parents and children. As much as a youth may want to return to the facility or a parent may beg you to come take their child back, it is important that family workers spend this time reaching out to the family. Help them work through these difficult times by helping them to learn to live together differently.

People live and change in the context of relationships (Fewster, 1990; Garfat, 1998; Krueger, 1998). Our work with youth and families focuses on how family members live in their relationships with each other. How people are with one another, the roles they adopt, the boundaries they maintain, and the care of their relationships are important to us. Relationships are in constant evolution, and family relationships change with time, circumstances, and events. This relationship evolution is a constant focus for the family worker because, as relationships evolve, so does the individual's experience of self and others. When you are with families where they live their lives, you are with them while they live their relationships.

These thoughts about relationship and process apply to all members of the family and to the relationship between the family and the family worker. Workers are also concerned with other relationships of importance that impact the family such as those with other professionals, community members, and extended family members. Sometimes attending to the process of relationship development is more important in helping a family to change than any specific content of discussion. Another historic pattern in many programs has been the assumption that "parents are the problem" (Fewster & Garfat, 1993; Garfat & McElwee, 2001). It is our belief that in many cases parents are the key to change. They know their child better than another professional ever could. Not tapping into this resource leaves huge gaps in the information we may need to aid in the interventions we suggest. We believe most parents are doing the best they can given their available information, knowledge, and skills. With this as a base, we work on providing more information and knowledge, teaching skills, and supporting parents to feel empowered to take control of the situations within their families that are difficult for them.

The fact that a child is "put into care" may appear to say clearly and loudly that the parents are not able to parent their child, even though this may not always be the case. The act of placement reinforces this perception for both child and family, making yet another obstacle for change. Ensuring that parents are consulted, empowered, and involved in every single step of life within a program helps to challenge that perception. Though we may question at times whether a parent is doing what is best for their child, in most cases what they are currently doing, their way of being together, is their best solution to their present difficulties (Durrant, 1993).

Although the saying, "it takes a village to raise a child" may seem simplistic, the root reflects the inclusiveness of systemic thinking.

It is essential to work systemically with youth and families, from using all resources from school, to friends, doctors, and other community resources in supporting change within families. Many of us have numerous experiences with youth who resided in our programs, apparently growing and changing in positive ways, only to go back home and return to the life that caused placement in the first place. We believe this is because families and other supports were not involved in the change process. Before working with families, you must develop a belief system and values that support families. Together these form a framework for a vision, and it is this vision that will guide a program in work with families. If this is not present and parents and their contributions are not valued, then change will not be successful, and parents will struggle to maintain involvement and confidence with the program.

It is important that these beliefs and values are clear prior to changing the program. It is essential that the supervisor talks with the team and that together they develop the framework to be used before embarking on working with families. In the end, some team members may not be in agreement with the philosophy that grows from the discussions and they may be left behind when it comes to working with parents and families either within or outside of the program.

NOT EVERYONE SHOULD DO THIS

As a supervisor, a major task is the creation of a strong team. When hiring, you look for specific qualities in youth workers. Of course they need skill and commitment with and to youth but also attributes that will complement and expand upon already established strengths within the team. This can be a difficult task, particularly for youth facilities located in smaller rural areas with fewer qualified individuals than in cities or towns with educational facilities that offer youth care programs or degrees.

Further, there are specific qualities that one must have to work with families that may or may not stand out when hiring someone to work only with youth. Some of these qualities cannot be easily identified in initial interviews and orientation. They are qualities that a supervisor must learn to look for, explore, and investigate as they get to know a particular youth care worker.

One skill that must be present is a highly defined ability to look at self in the context of work with youth and families (Ricks & Garfat, 1989). When working with families, this skill is important because you are dealing with issues that involve not only youth but men, women, mothers, fathers, and issues such as their relative place and role within the family as well as morality. That is why it essential that all youth workers do not automatically become family workers. When beginning the process of working with families, care and thought must be given to which workers within the program have the abilities and, most importantly, the fit and feel to work with parents and other family members. There are issues involved that might be viewed one way within the treatment milieu and quite differently within a family home. Drug use by youth and their families is a good example of an issue that illustrates how the work may have a different meaning in the context of a family.

In general, drug use by youth is something that is not accepted when working with youth in a residential facility. When a youth is a regular user of drugs, whatever the drug may be, it is usually tackled as an "issue." Within the program, there are tools that come into play when an issue is identified, which may include consequences, treatment plan goals, or more aggressive treatment tools such as drug counseling, rehabilitation programs, or law enforcement. Although occasional recreational drug use may be something that youth care workers chose to ignore, it is not routinely "left alone." Within the treatment program, this issue is generally not controversial or difficult for youth care workers or teams. The themes are relatively universal, and it is rare when disputes about dealing with drug issues arise.

Drug use within a family can be a completely different matter. There may be a need for workers to accept and not judge certain adult behaviors, particularly with adults whose behaviors directly effect the lives of their children. It may be necessary for workers to look past their individual views about drug use when working with parents.

The ability to accept value differences as well as the ability to separate out their own feelings on some issues is a key to building a relationship with a family member. Adults should make choices knowing the consequences of their actions. Even if this is not completely true, the focus must be encouraging change as it relates to the family and the goals set and not necessarily tackling an issue, even if we think the behavior is wrong. If a parent's drug use is peripheral to the goals designed with the family, it may not be wise to target it.

This and similar issues may lead to struggles by youth and family workers about what to address and what to leave alone. It is also an example of the type of issue that may separate those who "fit" with family work and those who do not. Some extremely skilled youth care workers may not have the "fit" to work with parents. This is when the struggle becomes that of the supervisor.

Families are systems, and all systems have rules and boundaries that those within the system follow. It is essential that we do not impose our rules on a family. This means we must be cautious not to judge the rules of the system but, instead, to look at those rules within the context of change. The behaviors that are supported by the family's boundaries and rules have meaning for the family and its members. In working with the family we must understand what the actions mean to and in the family. Part of our job might be to find out which rules are working for them and which ones are not.

When making the transition to family work, supervisors must assess the strengths of individual workers and mentally separate the team into those who are ready and those who are not ready. This separation can be reframed into "taking care of the floor," ensuring some workers maintain full attention to the day-to-day operation of the program. This may be easier said than done. Many workers see the transition to working with families as a promotion or advancement and, perhaps, in some way it is. It is an extension of the individual and group work with youth and brings the work of the program full circle.

In addition, the rewards are sometimes more easily seen. When working with youth, the payoff can be years down the road. Change within families can be more visible and may come more quickly. Further, adults are usually more comfortable than youth about giving workers feedback, whether positive and negative, which can be either gratifying or scary.

One way to lessen the possible negative impact of this differentiation between workers is to ensure that all team members—working with families or not—are supported and nurtured into tasks at which they are skillful. If family work is not the right fit, then it might be necessary to focus the worker in another direction whether that be life-skills, recreation, group work, or a different area in which they are interested and skilled. As you do this, you can also set up educational goals, trainings, and readings to help them gain the skills they need to do family work down the road. There are also other ways to ensure the workers not working with families continue to grow.

One good approach is to pair less experienced and less skilled workers with mentors. The less experienced worker's actual role within a case or family may be as simple as watching and talking with the key worker. This way they may see how the worker thinks and watch them interact with parents.

The family worker often becomes the closest help care provider the parent has ever experienced. In some ways the relationship may be more intimate than their relationships with doctors, therapists, or social workers. Because the family worker is on site within the family home, certain walls and barriers that families typically use are not possible, making it very scary at times, but also, because the worker is there with them through the struggle, safer.

Supervision is more difficult when work is done outside of the residential facility, because supervisors are not going to be with the worker all of the time, and because much of the work is done within the home. The level of trust between worker and supervisor is, therefore, that much more important.

The decision about who should or should not be doing this work is the first and maybe the most important part of the process a program undertakes when working with families. Training and additional learning about working with families is also essential before beginning. However, this does not always ensure that a youth care worker can work with families any more than a youth care degree can ensure a person is capable of work with youth. There are some youth care workers who, although wonderful with individual youth, struggle to deal effectively and respectfully with adults, whether that be parents or the team members they work with everyday.

THE APPROACH MAY BE THE SAME, BUT THE ACTIONS ARE DIFFERENT

A child and youth care approach can be easily transferred to working with families, but it may not encompass all areas that relate to family. Working with adults and families can be very different than individual work with youth.

The relationship between worker and family members possesses certain characteristics that define it is as different from most of the other relationships in the life of families. One of the most noticeable characteristics of the youth care helping relationship is that it is a relationship of intentionality (Garfat, 1998; Ricks & Garfat, 1989). The relationship exists only in order to support change and development in the family. Thus the actions of the worker are directed towards the development of the relationship for the purpose of facilitating change for the individuals involved in the relationship. In many cases, it is in the relationship with the worker that family members find the trust, support, and opportunity to try new ways of being or being together.

SCHEDULING FOR FAMILY WORK

OK, so you are now working with families. Great. Everyone is happy, the program is expanding, and you feel you are finally doing all you can to help youth and families. But Sally and Martin, your best workers, are now off the floor and in the homes of families for several hours a couple of times a week.

Without their strength on the floor other workers are feeling unsupported and without their safety net, and the youth are acting out accordingly. What now? Scheduling–good scheduling–is something many
people do not think about enough when beginning work with families or,
for that matter, any program development that takes workers off the floor.

Over the years most programs develop a careful balance about who is working, when they are working, and how. Supervisors are generally able to predict
when they will get the most calls and when they will get no calls. The strength
and consistency of the team are things that youth workers, supervisors, and
youth in particular come to expect. It is essential that as work with families
outside the residential facility begins, careful planning has taken place to ensure that workers and youth are not sent into a state of shock when some workers are not there as much as they used to be.

At Nexus, three workers are scheduled each evening. Two are expected to
be working the floor with the youth in residence as their primary responsibility. The third person works with families outside of the facility or sometimes
doing other tasks within the facility. This works well. However, it is not perfect, nor is it predictable. Crisis happens when it happens, and the youth/family
workers must be ready to be supportive when these crises occur. It is therefore
essential, when planning schedules, that the first priority be the facility program, and that the work with youth on the floor is not harmed. Youth and
workers should not feel that they are being sacrificed when another worker
juggles dual responsibilities. Therefore, one rule is that when working the
floor, work the floor! It is important that workers who have families on their
case load try as much as possible to plan their work with them around their
floor work and not try to juggle phone calls or visits during down time on the
floor shift. Youth need to know that the workers on shift are available for them,
as do the other youth workers working the floor. This is not to say that a particular worker may not be pulled away, but when possible a competent replacement worker should be provided who can contribute as much as the worker
who is being pulled away. Despite the demands of working with families, a
worker on the floor, particularly during a bad night, can be envious of the
worker driving off alone to spend time with families, leaving them feeling
abandoned and unsupported.

As family work begins, one of your most experienced and skilled part-time
workers should be sought out to fill in on a consistent basis for workers taken
off the floor. If this worker is respected and familiar to the team and the youth,
it may be seen as positive that the regularly scheduled worker is pulled off the
floor. This can be a great opportunity for a casual worker, and it means that the
worker leaving the program can focus on the tasks at hand and not have to
worry about what is going on back at the program.

The ideal is to schedule workers so that there are hours from the floor schedule that workers may spend with families. For example, with a 32-hour shift week and another eight hours of flexible time, the worker can use these for work with families without those on the floor being adversely affected. This is not perfect, but it does lessen the negative effect on the residential program as a whole. This method can be a challenge for workers, because it means some days off are not truly off. These hours must be inserted somewhere. Some workers may not be flexible, and close supervision may be needed so the worker does not accumulate a large backlog of hours owed to the agency.

Scheduling problems cannot be avoided. They can be reduced with planning and a skilled and large part-time worker pool. Yet one can never plan for all needs, and the goal is to have workers who are able to make the youth, workers in the facility, and the families outside of the building feel that they are the main priority when the worker is with them. It can be a struggle for individual workers to ensure that team members, youth, and families receive the attention they need. This struggle leads to stress if the proper planning is not done. Although some days off may be sacrificed for work responsibilities, others, including vacation days, must be untouchable so that the workers do not feel they are being pulled in all directions all of the time.

In addition to proper scheduling, it is important the worker be given time with the supervisor to discuss and reflect on the outside work. This is particularly important for family work, where immediate feedback is not readily available. Besides supervisor feedback, reflecting on the work during discussions with team members and at team meetings provides emotional release, an opportunity to problem solve, a place to regain balance, and it is a natural way to process achievement as well.

YOUR FAMILY VERSUS THEIR FAMILY

Families are an important and essential part of our work with youth, and our own families are usually the most important part of our lives. Work with families creates personal and scheduling conflicts that are reduced by knowing the schedule in advance and being able to plan personal lives around it.

Still, working with the families of others throws a big wrench into planning and predictability for their own lives, causing some workers to struggle. This is true especially for new parents or people with new partners in their lives. It is important that we attempt to reframe this change from a problem to an asset. As we strive toward professional standards, this flexibility is essential to the success. Lawyers, doctors, and other professionals adapt to the needs of the people they serve, and so must family workers. The strength of working with families from a youth care approach is the ability to work "in the moment." In our role as youth care professionals, we have stretched this term to "in the moment, we happen to be on shift." This is acceptable for floor work within the facility, because there are always other youth workers working when we are not on shift. With family work, this is not the case.

It is often necessary, particularly with families who are struggling, that youth care staff is available 24 hours a day, seven days a week. Family work cannot be rigidly scheduled. This does not mean that the worker's personal life must stop. It may mean that more than one worker is assigned to the family, so that someone is always able to be there when needed. We do not want to be crisis workers, however, and the best form of intervention is not always rushing when a family calls. With time and support, parents are more often than not capable of solving problems. It is important that all team members know what is going on within a family and are able to offer support even if that support is restricted to conversations over the phone. Families, like youth, do not need to know that someone will always come running, but they do need to know that someone is always there.

Because we have chosen to work with families in the context of their daily lives, and because we are committed to helping them learn to live their lives differently in the places where they live, we must be available: time and space. It is important to have the flexibility of staffing, program, and schedule to meet the needs of both worker and family.

When you are dealing with workers who may not be as available when not scheduled, it is more essential that additional supports be in place. No one should be expected to drop his or life for work every time there is a need. If appropriate schedule adjustments are made (e.g., an extra day off to balance times when the worker may be on call), then it should be possible for the worker to be available when needed. If this cannot be done, someone else should be ready to support a family if crisis arises. And most families say that the telephone conversations during a crisis, and most especially the times when team members just "spent time" with them, were the most valuable aspect of the work for them. Our role should be to facilitate answers, not to give solutions. Families have their own answers, it may just require someone to help them find them.

MONEY, MONEY, MONEY

When thinking about a new program, people often think their biggest difficulty is going to be coming up with the money. Obtaining new money, even for a worthwhile program, is not an easy task. Most governments do not grant additional funds to residential programs, even when it might save money in the long run. Fortunately, it is possible for a program to make the transition to working with families without requiring enormous quantities of additional cash. What is needed, as stated, is additional planning and, most importantly, the willingness to be flexible with time and scheduling.

When thinking about working with families it is most important to think creatively about the use of time. There are occasions in most programs when there is down time, whether that be throughout the day when youth are in programs or school, or on weekends when the in-house numbers may be lower. These are a good time to begin the transition to working with families. A youth care worker can drive a youth home and begin relationship building by visiting with the family at these times, and it may not add any costs while becoming a crucial part of success with a youth or family.

It is essential to take every opportunity to talk with parents. If they call to speak with their child, take some time before "calling Amy" to ask how they are, how their day went, if they watched the game last night. One of the main obstacles to building relationships with parents is their view that, somehow, professionals are people to be feared. Once this fear is reduced, many things can happen with families without a lot of effort or cost. Beginning work with families does not have to take additional funding. Working with families can be integrated into any program without affecting the budget significantly, though we do recognize that to make families a large part of the program can and does require additional money, at least at the beginning.

In some programs, work with families within the program is usually not billed as an additional cost. If you want to be able to bill for this work, you must first have a program in place to show to agencies and that validates the program with goals, desired outcomes, and a detailed plan of how the money will benefit the case, the youth and, since we are talking about budgets, the agency as well. With most issues involving money it is crucial to be able to show that spending the money will actually save money. Spending time with the family of the youth decreases a youth's time within residential care and reduces subsequent expenses. In advance, this can be difficult to sell, and it needs to be backed up with evidence.

Family members should experience success in their own environment. We want the satisfaction of success to be associated with home and family, not a professional's office. This does not always take additional money. Another inexpensive choice is if a worker is able to leave the floor for a short time without being replaced, then there is no cost for time with a parent or family.

Yet when a youth care worker leaves the floor to work with a family outside of the center, in most cases that worker does need to be replaced. This replacement cost is what we need to calculate when budgeting for family work. When a youth is referred and during your initial meetings with youth, parents, and the agency, workers assess how much time is needed per week in the home with the family and attempt to get these hours approved in the beginning. Many referring workers will approve additional funding for accompanying youth to doctor appointments, for anger management, drug counseling, and other program-related activities. We need to think of family work in the same manner: a part of the program necessary for success. It is important not to shy away from the role and authority that we have in residential care. If we are providing a service that is beneficial and successful, having more hours or additional funding approved may be easier than you think.

Another strategy for keeping initial costs low and for building an argument for additional funding is to begin with one youth and one family so you have a base of success from which to work. It may also be helpful to begin with your home agency or the agency with which you most closely work. If your work with one family is known throughout this agency, you may find the money is offered to you instead of having to ask.

Social workers and agencies want success as much as we do. It is what they see and hear, not necessarily what we say, that will lead to additional funding for these extra hours.

CONCLUSIONS

It has been our experience that many of the issues encountered in residential care come down to a youth's perception of him or herself, particularly in relation to family and parents. It is the family that helps create us, and it is in the family that we often find our greatest struggles.

When discussing a child with a parent, it is fascinating to see how the parents' struggles about their own parents somehow reappear with their own child. It is difficult to imagine how concentrating solely on one family member will lead to lasting change within the family as a whole, as a system. We talk about Susan, for example, and remember when her older brother Richard was here.

It should be noted that these ideas are a designed approach. The full approach within the Nexus program is not just one person's values and beliefs but is made up of those who were there before and those of the team who were present when the approach was adopted. Some who worked at Nexus at the time may or may not have fully supported it. Some have left–some remain. Newer workers have come to Nexus and some have fully supported it, although some have not. Some work with families–some do not. It is our approach; we believe it is right for us. Your approach when deciding to work with families must come from the values, beliefs, and shared experience and knowledge of those who will be acting on them in their work with families. Anything less, or anything not fully supported, will not succeed.

Since we began working with families, success has been clearly visible. Having something so clearly beneficial was new to our team, because success in residential care was often difficult and almost impossible to see. We tended to measure our success by what a social worker might tell us or, most importantly, the visits or calls from residents who left the program years earlier.

Working with families also increases the amount of service a program is able to provide, without significant increases in cost. You can have a full building yet still work with a family, because the two are not always interconnected. Nexus has six long-term and two emergency beds. The clearest form of success for us is that we now work with almost 20 youth, not just eight, and when you include families, the numbers are close to 100. One hundred people are supported, in contrast to six or eight, by the same number of youth and family workers. In addition, this makes possible admitting youth into our family program, youth who in the past would have moved directly into residential care but now can remain at home with supports for them and their parents. This consequence is truly rewarding.

Families need our support, more often so than individual youth. The youth is sometimes seen as the problem, not just because of their actions but because of what these actions and this child mean to the parents. All actions serve a purpose. If, for example, a child's actions are to get attention from a parent, helping the child see that is only half the battle. The parents must see it as well and learn different ways to meet the needs of their children.

REFERENCES

Durrant, M. (1993). *Residential treatment: a cooperative, competency-based approach to therapy and program design*. New York: W. W. Norton.

Fewster, G. (1990). *Being in child care: a journey into self*. New York: The Haworth Press, Inc.

Fewster, G., & Garfat, T. (1993). Residential child and youth care. In C. Denholm, R. Ferguson, & A. Pence (Eds.), *Professional child and youth care* (2nd ed., pp. 9-36).Vancouver, BC: University of British Columbia Press.

Garfat, T. (1998). The effective child and youth care intervention. *Journal of Child and Youth Care, 12*, 1-178.

Garfat, T., & McElwee, N. (2001). The changing role of family in child and youth care practice. *Journal of Child and Youth Care Work, 15-16*, 236-248.

Krueger, M. (1998). *Interactive youth work practice*. Washington, DC: Child Welfare League of America.

Ricks, F., & Garfat, T. (1989). Working with individuals and their families: considerations for child and youth care workers. *Journal of Child and Youth Care Work, 5*(1), 63-70.

Index

Acting with purpose, 59
Active self-awareness, child and youth
    care practice and, 12
Activity, 134–135
    care-taking roles and, 143
    encouragement in, 140
Activity programming, 134–135
    for child and youth care practice,
      135–139
    in family-focused child and youth
      care practice, 141–144
    implementing, into family-focused
      child and youth care practice,
      139–141
    life space, 140
Addams, Jane, xxi,xxii,xxiii
Advocacy
    interventions and, 109–110
    teaching, 104–105
Analogue work, 73

Beliefs, for working with families,
    212–214
Biological family, 2
Boundaries, 69, 74,88–89,216

Calgary Board of Education, 96
Calgary Catholic Family Services, 96
Calgary Health Region, 96
Caregiving, person's history of, 26–27
Caretaker models
    multiple, 139
    primary, 138–139
Care-taking roles, and activity, 143
Care workers. *See* Child and youth
    care workers

Catholic Family Services (Calgary,
    Alberta), 96
Change, 108–109
    case study of, 97–107
    creating lasting, 81–82
    development stages of client and,
      113–114
    pain and, 102–103
    process of, 102
    relationships and, 112,213
    taking long-term view of, 99
Child and youth care approach, xxii.
    See also Ethical practice;
      Ireland;
      Residential care programs
    "active self-awareness" and, 12
    activity-oriented, 141–144
    activity programming for, 135–139
    articulating, 82
    assumptions about, 9–13
    case study of, 8–9,32–36
    challenges of involving families in,
      173–175
    changes in family involvement and
      work in, 4,5t
    characteristics of, 217
    characteristics of interventions of,
      14–24
    caring for family and family
      members, 14–16
    family fit and, 19–24
    immediacy and connected to
      goals, 16–19
    constructing relationships in,
      198–199
    daily events for therapeutic
      purposes and, 12–13
    details of family living and, 43
    families and, 69–70,105–106

Values
  conflicts with, for child and youth
    care workers, 50
  incorporating family, 43–44

Youth. *See* Children
Youth care practice. *See* Child and
    youth care approach
Youth family workers. *See* Child and
    youth care workers
Youth workers. *See* Child and youth
    care workers